Deafness and Education in the UK
Research Perspectives

D0817244

Deafness and Education in the UK
Research Perspectives

Edited by

Clare Gallaway PhD, MA (Lond), DipTEO (Manchester)
Editor, Deafness and Education International
Formerly Senior Lecturer in Education
University of Manchester

and

Alys Young PhD, MSc (Oxon), BA (Cantab)
Senior Lecturer in Deafness and Deaf Education,
University of Manchester

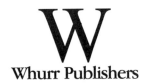

Whurr Publishers

Chapter 3 © M. Mahon
© all other material 2003 Whurr Publishers Ltd
First published 2003
by Whurr Publishers Ltd
19b Compton Terrace
London N1 2UN
England

British Library Cataloguing in Publication Data

A catalogue record for this book is available from the British Library.

ISBN 1 86156 369 8

Typeset by Adrian McLaughlin, a@microguides.net
Printed and bound in the UK
by Athenæum Press Ltd, Gateshead, Tyne & Wear.

Contents

Research Trust, is the ascertainment study which identified more than 17 000 deaf children born between 1980 and 1997 in the UK (Fortnum et al, 2002). The advent of screening of newborn infants for hearing throughout the UK, just beginning as this volume is being prepared, is yet another initiative which will undoubtedly provide the impetus for research.

There are some particular reasons for the emergence of a research community in the UK during the 1990s. In no small measure, three sets of Research Seminar Series funded by the Economic and Social Research Council played a role in allowing researchers in deafness to meet, share approaches, and share and benefit from work carried out by eminent researchers from overseas. The 1993 series led by Ruth Campbell (University College, London) and the 1996/97 series led by John Clibbens (University of Plymouth) were concerned with deafness and cognition, but even in the first series, the relevance of this chiefly psychology-based research to deaf children's education was clearly outlined by Campbell in a guest editorial (Campbell, 1996). In the second series, Clibbens remarks that although the seminars were research-led, discussion of applications was prominent (Clibbens, 1998). In the third set, led by Susan Gregory (University of Birmingham) the topic of the seminars was now defined as Deafness and Education. Further research meetings continued at Birmingham (DERG: the Deafness and Education Research Group), and in the North West (NOWCORD: the North West Consortium of Researchers in Deafness.)

The importance of these meetings cannot be overestimated. These opportunities to meet on a national and multidisciplinary basis and to have access to presentations from overseas scholars, particularly from the US, lent coherence to the UK research community. A further boost to research was the inauguration of two new academic research journals in 1996: the *Journal of Deaf Studies and Deaf Education* (US) and *Deafness and Education*, subsequently *Deafness and Education International* (UK). Until then, there was no real national publication platform for research carried out in the UK. The British Association of Teachers of the Deaf and Whurr Publishers combined to produce the first UK academic journal in this area. Papers given at the Seminar Series and reports of the meetings have been included at first in *JDSDE,* and more recently also in *DEI.*

This volume has been designed to cover a wide range of UK research which concerns the education and development of deaf children. Most is not what would be termed 'educational research'; rather, it draws on a wide variety of disciplines and their differing research paradigms. It is important to note also the increase in the number of deaf academics and deaf research students in the UK, and the volume reflects the growth in involvement of deaf people in educational research and practice. Some of the research reported also highlights the impact of new medical and scientific technologies on educational research with deaf children.

The contents include some reference to educational settings over the whole age range, early years education, primary and secondary classrooms, children in family and clinical settings as well as in school, and work with students in both further and higher education. Some chapters report as yet undisseminated work, whereas other chapters survey known work, albeit of current import. Both large-scale and small-scale studies are included, as well as surveys, case studies and work from a range of educational settings. Contributors include both deaf and hearing researchers, both widely published and less experienced writers, and are from a range of disciplines: language and linguistics, education, social science, audiology, and psychology.

However, this selection of chapters is in no way definitive. It is intended rather as a snapshot, indicative of what is going on in the UK. Many other researchers and research teams could have been included, and indeed it would now be quite possible to design another, similar, volume which would include important work and both senior and junior researchers omitted from this one.

The chapters have been grouped according to theme and each section contains a commentary which draws together the chapters within it. Some chapters also contribute to the themes of other sections. For instance, Hopwood's study is concerned with language analysis and also support for learning; Archbold and Nikolopoulos are also concerned with measuring attainments.

The first section, 'Interaction at Home and at School', is a well-visited theme for education and child development in general and the five chapters in it visit different aspects of early environment and development. In Part 2, 'Focusing on Progress and Attainment', there are three chapters concerned with very different aspects of deaf children's education within the school context. Thirdly, 'Support for Learning' deals with the mechanics of what is provided for deaf children and students to access the curriculum, either by way of assistive devices or by 'scaffolding' within the classroom context to facilitate learning.

Preface

In research and academic study, edited collections of research papers are now commonplace and, some might say, have become an essential resource. Indeed it is our impression that in some fields, edited collections are beginning to outnumber books written by individual authors. These volumes may arise from papers given at a conference, or they may simply be the editors' response to a complex, multidisciplinary field, by inviting a number of scholars each to write about their own work.

This edited volume is the first – and, we hope, not the last – collection of papers about deafness and education research to be published in the UK. For many years, UK scholars and professionals have turned to the wealth of substantial and useful texts produced in the United States, and undoubtedly will continue to do so. However, although our research must be of an international standard, there is of course a need for it to deal with local conditions. For instance, it needs to encompass specific features, such as the nature of education offered to deaf children in British services, the use of British Sign Langauage (BSL) in the classroom, and the extent and quality of technical, scientific and medical resources available in the UK.

It is pleasing that it is at last possible to produce such a book based on research carried out in the UK. Ten years ago, this would have been difficult to do. When planning this book, we were aware that it would be possible within a very short timescale to plan another similar volume by inviting a range of different colleagues. This is very encouraging, but should not lead to complacency. We have made progress, but not enough. We firmly believe that a sound knowledge base gained through research is an essential cornerstone of progress; the relationship between research findings and practical applications is complex, however, and there must be continuing dialogue both across disciplines and also between academics and professionals.

To acknowledge all those who have contributed in some way to the completion of this book would be impossible. However, the first thanks must of course go to all the chapter authors for their hard work in producing careful and interesting contributions.

Our thanks also to Judith Nugent who has provided excellent administrative support in the production of this volume.

Above all, we are indebted to the research community: in particular, those who have dedicated uncounted hours labouring to organize day and weekend seminars, and those who have steadfastly attended such meetings even in the face of transport difficulties, lack of funding and overwork. We would also like to extend a warm vote of thanks to scholars from overseas who have been happy to visit and support our meetings and by so doing, have generally encouraged and inspired our own efforts.

We trust that this book will prove to be a useful text to both researchers and practitioners alike and will contribute to a better understanding of how to enable deaf children to achieve the potential that is rightly theirs.

Clare Gallaway
Alys Young

Contributors

Sue Archbold
Nottingham Paediatric Cochlear Implant Programme
Clare Gallaway
Editor, *Deafness and Education International*
Mary Griggs
Centre for Deaf Studies, University of Bristol
Frank Harrington
Department of Education and Social Science (Deaf Studies),
University of Central Lancashire
Peter Hindley
National Deaf Services, London
Vicky Hopwood
York Consulting, Leeds
Ailsa Laidler
City College Manchester
Julian Lloyd
Human Communication and Deafness, University of Manchester
Wendy McCracken
Human Communication and Deafness, University of Manchester
Merle Mahon
Human Communication Science, University College London
Christine Merrell
Curriculum, Evaluation and Management Centre, University of
Durham
Thomas Nikolopoulos
Nottingham Paediatric Cochlear Implant Programme
Rachel O'Neill
City College Manchester
Meg Shepherd
Wrexham Maelor Hospital, Wales

Hilary Sutherland
Freelance research consultant
Ruth Swanwick
School of Education, University of Leeds
Granville Tate
Curriculum, Evaluation and Management Centre, University of Durham
Noel Traynor
School of Nursing, University of Salford
Peter Tymms
Curriculum, Evaluation and Management Centre, University of Durham
Alys Young
Human Communication and Deafness, University of Manchester

PART 1
INTERACTION AT HOME AND AT SCHOOL

Commentary

CLARE GALLAWAY AND ALYS YOUNG

The young child's path to adulthood is based on cognitive and social development, which can only take place through interaction with others and with the environment. In particular, language develops through interaction. Children acquire their language, or languages, largely in and through conversations with others. Language is not merely a vehicle for thoughts and a tool for learning but is also inextricably bound up with a person's identity and role, as perceived both by self and by others. Infants in the early years embark on a long journey of discovery and learning – how to be adults and members of the society around them. This journey begins in the home but across the childhood years, development in the home context is increasingly complemented by development in the classroom, not all of which is of a formal nature.

The context for the infant's earliest learning is the home and the family. For young deaf children and those caring for them, there are some key issues to be considered. One is that professionals are likely to be involved closely with infants and their families from the earliest point, and intervention to facilitate the pre-school deaf child's development takes place in a home or clinic setting. An increasingly common type of intervention is described by Sutherland, Griggs and Young in Chapter 1, where an account is given of family intervention projects in the UK involving deaf adults. Deaf children are most often born into hearing families, so that no deaf adult is in the child's immediate surroundings, and the hearing parents also are likely to have little experience or understanding of deafness. The introduction of deaf adults into the child's life, therefore, can have a number of beneficial effects at an early stage. The research reported here was part of a much-needed comprehensive survey of such intervention projects in the UK.

A priority for deaf infants and children is to ensure that their chances of developing language are maximized. An adequate and age-appropriate

1

language system is a prerequisite to successful learning and the difficulties many young deaf children experience with acquiring a full language system are well known. The context and course of early communicative and language development in hearing children has been systematically and extensively researched for four decades now but in comparison, developmental accounts of deaf children's early language and the contexts of interaction are still rather sparse. In particular, developmental accounts and detailed analyses of actual interaction are not widespread. There are several obvious and unavoidable reasons why this is so.

Since profound childhood deafness presents an obstacle to language development, research funding and general attentional effort towards deaf children is generally geared to facilitating their development. Also, access to deaf infants and young children as subjects for observational and experimental research in language development is extremely limited – either because infants are already suffering a surfeit of professional attention, or because the professional bodies charged with their care may not wish or be able to allow access to researchers. Ethically, this seems understandable, but it means that whereas in mainstream language development research there is a vast bank of data, description and analysis, for deaf children there is very little.

The remaining chapters in this section are all concerned with different and particular aspects of language interaction with deaf children. They all provide some information in areas which are virtually unresearched so far. Two consider the family setting (Shepherd and Gallaway, Mahon) and two are concerned with the educational setting (Lloyd, Hopwood).

Polyadic interaction – that is, conversations involving more than two people – has not been widely researched, but within the family it is generally common to have more than two participants in a conversation. Shepherd and Gallaway's chapter presents a fine-grained analysis of interaction within a family, exploring conversations between a 2-year-old deaf child and different groupings of the members of his (hearing) family. Their analysis is concerned with defining different parental and sibling styles and considering how far the interaction may be helpful to the child's language-learning processes.

Many millions of the world's children grow up in a multilingual environment. Deaf children may be educated or reared bilingually with spoken and signed language both playing a role. However, many deaf children will also grow up in settings where two or more spoken languages are available. Mahon's chapter is concerned with deaf children in homes where the language of the home is Sylheti and English is an additional language. For her study of 7-year-olds and their parents, she uses a conversation analysis (CA) framework to focus on question–answer sequences. She considers how far appropriate language learning opportunities are being provided and what implications this may have for choice of spoken language with a deaf child in a bilingual family.

Another little-researched area is the interaction between deaf and hearing children of school age. Lloyd points out that increasingly, with policies of inclusion, deaf children are being taught alongside their hearing peers. However, the benefits of integration for deaf children have not been clearly demonstrated in the research literature, and Lloyd's study considers some ways in which learning alongside hearing children may be beneficial to deaf children's language development. The framework is one of structured communication tasks, where children's competence as speakers and listeners is tested. This study is concerned with the evaluation of spoken language skills but the framework could be easily applied to further similar investigations such as competence in communicating in total communication classrooms, as Lloyd points out.

Hopwood similarly found no earlier research looking at features of interaction within different support situations in the classroom. She points out that 80% of deaf children in the UK are thought to be being educated through spoken language within the mainstream, and that this often entails a variety of staff providing support via spoken language. Like Mahon, she has focused on question–answer sequences, but has used a framework of that was devised originally to analyse classroom interaction. Subtle differences in question–answer sequences may be found when a fine-grained analysis is applied and the implications for language development are discussed.

Chapter 1
Deaf adults and family intervention projects

Hilary Sutherland, Mary Griggs and Alys Young

Background

Family intervention projects explicitly designed to employ deaf adults to work with hearing families with deaf children are becoming more common. Projects are reported in countries as diverse as the USA (Watkins, Pitman and Walden, 1998), Scandinavia (Drasgow, 1993), Israel (Dromi and Ingber, 1999), Australia (Mohay et al, 1998), Germany (Hintermair, 2000), The Netherlands (van der Lem, 1987) and the UK (Sutherland and Kyle, 1983). Although the structures of these projects often vary considerably, three underlying aims commonly recur:

- **To introduce parents to a deaf[1] adult who is a positive role model.** For many hearing parents with deaf children, what it is to be deaf is hard to imagine and the vast majority will never have met a deaf person (Gregory, 1976). Through being given the opportunity to meet a deaf adult, parents gain an experience of deafness from the perspective of someone who is also deaf. They are able to ask questions about what it is like to be a deaf child and what kinds of lives deaf adults enjoy. Seemingly trivial worries such as: can deaf people drive? do deaf people marry? can be immediately resolved. Negative stereotypes about deafness are challenged through the immediate relationship with someone who is deaf. In essence, the approach works on an assumption of 'seeing is believing'. Parents given such opportunities for sustained and planned contact with a

---

[1] Conventionally upper case 'D' is used to designate references to cultural Deafness/Deaf people and lower case 'd' for references to those who would not identify themselves in this way, but we have not used this distinction in this chapter. In most cases projects were indeed working with 'D'eaf role models, but this was not always so, and also not all children involved necessarily had at that time in their development a self-acknowledged 'D'eaf identity.

deaf adult have reported feeling more relaxed about having a deaf child (Svartholm, 1993) and less anxious about their parental role (Hintermair, 2000). In projects that work with older deaf children, deaf adults act as role models for the children also, modelling, for example, strategies for independence and confident communication in unfamiliar environments (Young, Sutherland and Griggs, 1999).

- **To encourage the use of Sign Language and/or other forms of signed communication within the family.** The deaf adults who work with families in these projects are usually Sign Language (e.g. BSL) users. They encourage parents and siblings to learn and use Sign Language in the family through games, deliberate 'teaching' (Hoffmeister and Shettle, 1981; Takala, Kuusela and Takala, 2000), and also through the natural circumstances of parents and children just having to interact with a deaf person (Bouvet, 1990). In the early years, it is often the visuality of language rather than a grasp of the fully grammatical Sign Language that is important. For example, parents explore with deaf adults the visual possibilities of signed communication (Young, 1997), acquire useful signed vocabulary, and learn how to structure their own communication routines so that the child attends to the language used (Mohay, 2000).

- **To expose families to the 'cultural model' of deafness and the deaf community.** Through these projects, parents typically are introduced to the notion that deafness can be a positive attribute rather than a disability and are provided with information about and experiences associated with the deaf community's own cultural norms (Sutherland, 1994). These can range from, at a basic level, learning deaf ways of attracting attention and deaf appropriate forms of touch, to a more sophisticated understanding of deaf traditions, cultural values and the organization and structure of the deaf community (Sutherland and Kyle, 1993). The approach stands in sharp contrast to other interventions that encompass an approach to deafness based on the assumption that it is a medical condition requiring repair and cure. In the case of some family support programmes, this contrast of a medical with a cultural model of deafness is not presented as an either/or experience to families, but rather as part of a menu of possibilities from which parents can draw in exploring the implications of deafness for their family (Young, 2001).

At the heart of these kinds of projects is not simply the employment of professionals who are deaf. Rather it is the identification and deliberate, positive exploitation of a 'deaf role' in interventions with families. This role encompasses a range of functions, skills and approaches to working with hearing families that are inherent to, and a direct consequence of, being deaf.

The situation in the UK

In the UK, a number of deaf adult intervention projects developed rapidly from the mid-1980s. The two most publicized were the 'Deaf Children at Home Project' in Bristol (Sutherland and Kyle, 1993) and the Deaf Instructor Team in Leeds (Knight, 1997) although others are known to have existed in Suffolk, Devon, Blackburn, Cumbria and Lincolnshire.

Although some of these developments have made links with others, projects have largely developed in isolation from each other. The deaf adults who work for them have never met on a national basis – a fact that stands in sharp contrast to deaf people working in mental health services who have access to the national organization 'Deaf Professionals in Mental Health'. Common training needs between projects have never been coordinated, with different services usually making their own arrangements. Consequently, the experience and knowledge gained from project innovation is rarely recycled in new project developments. Evaluations of the impact of these projects is scarce and usually remains internal to that service, meaning that comparisons between service arrangements have never been made. From the parents' perspective, it is actually difficult to discover where such projects exist if they wish to have access to them as there is no national picture available.

In addition, although these services significantly share similar aims and characteristics, they are not necessarily funded or organized in a similar way. Some have received funding from charitable organizations, others operate under the auspices of Education Authorities, Social Services Departments and in some cases, of large deaf-related organizations such as the National Deaf Children's Society (NDCS) (*http://www.ndcs.org.uk*) and the Royal National Institute for Deaf People (RNID) (*http://www.rnid.org.uk*). The effects (both positive and negative) of such different funding arrangements, lines of service accountability, and varying characteristics of multi-agency working and responsibility have never been evaluated.

Research aims

It was in response to these significant gaps in our knowledge about deaf adult family intervention projects in the UK that the following research study was undertaken. The study had five aims:

- To produce a comprehensive national survey (for England and Wales) of family intervention projects using deaf adult role models that identified the location, aims, target populations and working arrangements of such projects.

- To investigate the effects of variations in funding arrangements, structural organization, and multi-professional contexts on the development and delivery of deaf adult family intervention projects.
- To collate information on the pre-existing evaluations of such projects.
- To analyse the characteristics of the employment of deaf adults in these projects.
- To evaluate the scope for joint working and joint service development between projects.

Design of the study

The fundamental problem facing the research was the location of the relevant projects in the first place. The study, therefore, used a two-phase survey design (full details in Young, Griggs and Sutherland, 2000). The first phase was aimed at identifying generally where deaf adults were working to support deaf children in any role or setting in England and Wales. The second was aimed at differentiating between two categories of respondent:

- Category A: Some of the employees in the service/project are deaf themselves, e.g. teachers and classroom assistants who are deaf, social workers who are deaf.
- Category B: The project/service was specifically set up to employ deaf people as service providers for families with deaf children, e.g. language aide projects, deaf home visitor projects, language links projects, etc.

Respondents self-selected which category best fitted their service and filled in a detailed questionnaire accordingly. The response rate to the phase 1 survey was 73.2% ($n = 568$) and to the phase 2 survey 62% ($n = 179$).

This chapter is concerned with the so-called Category B projects, but detailed information is available on the 131 Category A returns as well (Young, Griggs and Sutherland, 2000).

Project location and maturity

We identified 36 projects in England and Wales that were specifically set up to employ deaf adults as role models working with deaf children and their families, and which were strongly characterized by the aims and underlying philosophy previously outlined. In a sense, this absolute figure was of less importance than the underlying pattern we found of growth and development of such projects over time. If the establishment of new projects is tracked over the 10-year period between 1988 (the first established project) and 1998–99 (the end point of this research study), two distinct peaks emerge demonstrating an increase in new projects:

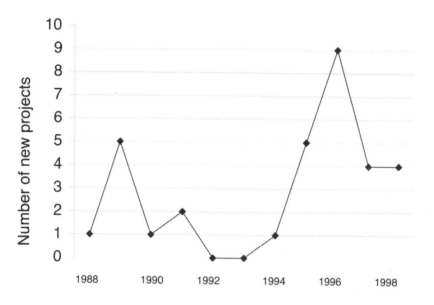

Figure 1.1 Project maturity – number of new projects established by year.

The peak in 1989 interestingly coincides with the Children Act (HMSO, 1989) which specifically allowed for the inclusion of deaf children within its newly designated category of 'children in need'. It also established the obligation of Local Authority Social Services Departments to consider and meet the needs of children thus defined – needs that according to the Act could encompass disadvantage arising from linguistic and cultural circumstances (Young and Huntington, 2002). Certainly one of the projects established at that time exploited this connection between 'children in need' as defined by the Act and the potential linguistic and cultural identity of deaf children in order to gain funding to establish itself. It may well be that others did the same.

The second peak in 1996 is more difficult to explain, but this was the year which saw the Education Act 1996 and the introduction of the Code of Practice attached to that Act which represented a legal obligation to provide for the needs of the child, which may include social, cultural and linguistic needs. Projects may have been set up to meet this recognized need.

If the cumulative number of projects in existence year on year is considered, then the dramatic scale and rate of growth becomes apparent. The actual number of projects in existence more than doubled between 1995–96 (15 projects) and 1998–99 (32 projects).

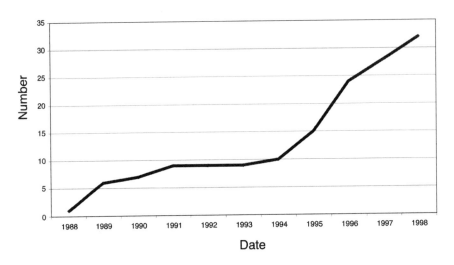

Figure 1.2 Cumulative number of projects in existence year by year.

Clearly this history of growth does not necessarily predict future trends. However, other available evidence does point to the likelihood, at least in the short term, of continued growth. First, the funding base of these projects is expanding as different agencies become more involved in resourcing projects (see section below). Second, the survey identified a further 12 respondents who were either seeking to set up such a project in the near future or who until recently had employed deaf adults to work with families. However, as discussed below, set against these positive markers of likely expansion, is a significant concern over short-term funding of new projects.

Project funding

The vast majority of projects (32 out of 36) were funded by a single source – education authority, social services or voluntary sector funding either through deaf organizations such as NDCS and/or as a result of a charitable grant, from Children in Need or The National Lottery for example. In a sense, this picture of predominantly single-agency funding was surprising. Deaf children and their families use a wide range of services with many different professionals cooperating to provide a network of support, greater joint funding of family intervention projects using deaf adult role models could perhaps have been expected, as multiple agencies would be likely to perceive an advantage in such arrangements.

However, it is worth noting that three out of the four projects that were actually funded jointly had been established within the last 3 years (during the period of rapid growth of projects) and this may indicate a trend towards greater joint funding in the future. Also a lack of joint funding does not necessarily imply lack of inter-agency cooperation. From other comments by respondents, it is clear that such cooperation does exist over such matters as referral mechanisms, supervision and project evaluation.

Of the 32 projects deriving their funding from a single source, education authorities had overall the biggest role, funding 16 of them (in addition to having a stake in three out of the four jointly-funded projects). Social services alone funded 9 projects. The other 7 were funded by either The National Lottery Charities Board or Children in Need, indicating more than a one-off commitment by these charities to this kind of approach to working with deaf children and their families.

Once again, however, it is the underlying trend rather than the overall picture that is more informative about the development of such projects. In the case of funding arrangements, if the post-1995 period (in which the number of projects doubled) is considered separately, then the picture is very different. Social services have a far greater stake in funding and education authorities a much smaller involvement in new projects.

It is unclear from the data available why these changes in ownership and funding of projects should be taking place and what the long-term consequences will be. It is, however, an important issue to consider for the future with the introduction of universal newborn hearing screening in England (*http://www.unhs.org.uk*) and its consequent impact on services. These services will be required to work with deaf babies and their families at a far younger age than had previously been common (RNID/NDCS, 2000).

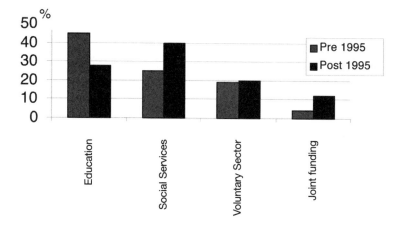

Figure 1.3 Comparison of funding arrangements before and after 1995.

Finally in relation to funding, it should be noted that securing the continuation and expansion of funding were significant concerns. Out of 10 developmental priorities, the securing of more funding and the retention of funding were ranked fourth and fifth respectively (behind encouraging more families to use the project, better training for deaf staff, and evaluation of the impact of the project). The increased role of charitable funding over the past 3 years in the expansion of project numbers also raises questions about short-termism, and how projects will survive after the life of the grant. It is known that some projects that have been established for a long time (such as those in Bristol and Leeds) have successfully become integrated into statutory service provision and are routinely available to families. How those transitions are made, however, and what influences the development from short-term project to ongoing provision remains largely unknown.

Age of children targeted by projects

Information on the age of the children was available for 27 out of the 36 projects. As expected, most ($n = 21$; 78%) incorporated work with pre-school deaf children, but in the case of only 3 projects were the early years an exclusive focus of intervention. The vast majority worked with a very wide age range of children, with half of the projects working with children of pre-school age right up to children in their mid to late teens.

In other words, project specialization in a particular developmental stage for children or in a particular period of adjustment for parents was

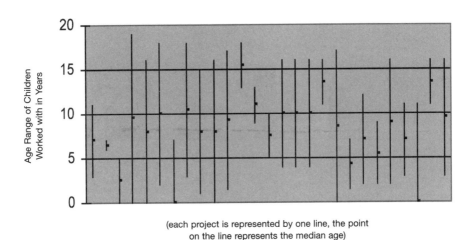

(each project is represented by one line, the point
on the line represents the median age)

Figure 1.4 Age of children in each project.

rare. This perhaps would not be a problem if projects themselves had many staff and where it could be imagined that some had particular expertise with particular family circumstances or age groups of children. (After all, there is a huge difference in acting as a role model for families when the deaf child is 2 and when the child is 14.) But the reality for these projects was that over half of them were staffed by only one person (see section on employment patterns, pp. 16–17). Therefore, it was more commonly the case that one deaf employee sought to meet the highly variable needs of children and families across a wide age span. This pattern is suggestive of pressure on projects to respond to whatever constituency of deaf children exists in a particular area, rather than projects planned and funded to meet specific developmental needs. Some evidence of such a trend has been previously documented (Young, Sutherland and Griggs, 1999).

In 34 out of the 36 projects, it was possible to identify how many families the projects had worked with since they were established. Not surprisingly, projects that had worked with the greatest number of families were the ones that had been established the longest. All of the 9 projects that had worked with 40 families or over had been established for at least 5 years.

Interestingly, the relationship between number of families worked with and length of time the project had been established did not hold true for those projects that had worked with the least number of families. Of the 12 projects that had worked with fewer than 10 families, 7 had been established for 3 or more years and 1 for nearly 10 years. These results might be explained by a range of factors: for instance, there might be variation in both the intensity and the duration of contact with families across projects.

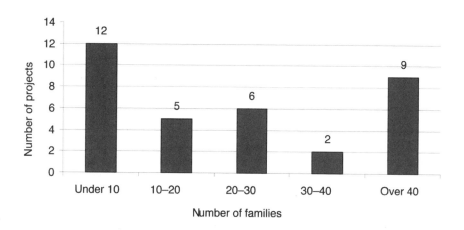

Figure 1.5 Number of families involved since projects started ($n = 34$)

Pattern of contact and project setting

Clearly the capacity of a given project for working with children and families is dependent on the number of personnel involved, but also on the pattern of contact and the settings in which the intervention takes place. Are children seen on an individual or group basis? Do families receive a time-bounded service or is contact open-ended? Also some projects might have single or multiple patterns of service delivery – working with children and families in a variety of ways. Considerable diversity was revealed about these issues from the 27 projects that were able to supply detailed information. The following discussion is presented in terms of 'categories of service delivery', because the 27 projects generated 32 instances of service delivery (Table 1.1), with 5 projects being involved in more than one activity e.g. a home visiting service *and* a school-based deaf children's group.

Table 1.1 Categories of service delivery described by projects

Category of service delivered by projects	Number of instances of each type of service category
Fixed in school timetable	7 (22%)
Flexible school based	7 (22%)
Flexible home based	2 (6%)
Weekly visits to child/family (blocks)	9 (28%)
Weekly visits to child/family (open ended)	3 (9%)
Weekly families' support group	1 (3%)
Monthly families' support group	1 (3%)
Respite care	2 (6%)
Total	32

Home- and family-based services

Of the 32 services reported by the projects, 14 (44%) were exclusively home-based – that is to say, deaf adults visit deaf children and their families in the home setting. Typically, families were worked with on an individual basis with 'family' including brothers and sisters, and in some cases extended family also.

Around two-thirds ($n = 9$) of these exclusively home-based projects worked with children and families according to a time-bounded pattern. Projects offered families a fixed number of sessions, usually based around a weekly pattern of visits. In some cases a specific number of sessions constituted one 'block' of material that children and families covered with their deaf home visitor. Families could then go on to receive further blocks. A detailed rationale for why, how and when parents should receive further contact from the deaf home visitor once the initial sessions were completed lay outside the scope of this study.

However, it would be an important subject to pursue further to gain a fuller understanding of how child/family need is determined and the basis on which it is met.

The other five examples of a home-based service were far less defined. Three operated an entirely open-ended approach to working with families. There was no predetermined number of contact visits nor any limit on how long a child/family could have contact with a project. The other two, described in Table 1.1 as 'flexible home based' were responsive services, offering home visits from deaf staff in accordance with a particular identified need at any given time. They were not fixed or predetermined intervention schemes.

It might be tempting to think that these less defined approaches to home based intervention were the newest projects, but this was not the case. In fact, the opposite was true, in that four of the these five projects were set up over 10 years ago. One explanation for this finding could be that the longer-established projects felt more confident in judging the need for intervention and, therefore, left contact open-ended. It may also be that patterns of service delivery established at the onset of the project have remained in place over the years. Larger projects are also more likely to have greater and more secure resources and might therefore be less likely to need to 'ration' intervention.

There were also two projects which in addition to their usual pattern of work, ran family support groups for hearing parents of deaf children (and in one case for grandparents of deaf children also). These took place outside the home setting and not everyone who attended was also receiving individual home visits.

There were also two projects that in a different sense were 'home-based' but fell outside the usual pattern of specially trained deaf adults visiting deaf children and hearing families at home. These two services were set up to provide respite care, i.e. the deaf child left the hearing family home and spent time in a deaf home/sign language environment. This respite care was designed both to provide linguistic/cultural enrichment for the children and to give parents a break from whatever strains they might be experiencing in bringing up their deaf child. The first project offered families a regular pattern of 1 day per week respite care, and the second offered families up to 28 days per year in a flexible/needs-led pattern.

School-based services

In addition to the home- or family-based services, there were 14 examples of school-based services provided by projects. Some of these were well-established services that had a fixed place in the school timetable. An example of this kind of service was a group run exclusively by deaf staff who come into the school to do so. They provide an environment in which deaf children can be totally immersed in BSL, in which only deaf adults and deaf children are present and in which children are encouraged to develop their deaf cultural identity.

Other examples of school-based services included regular contact between a deaf adult and children in a classroom setting to support the children's learning, and that was a fixed part of the school timetable. There were also more flexible versions of this kind of activity – where a deaf adult worked with a child as the need arose at any given time. At first glance it is difficult to distinguish these kinds of activity from instances in which deaf people are more straightforwardly employed as classroom assistants. Nonetheless, respondents described themselves as Category B projects instead of – or as well as – Category A services. Why respondents did so, and what seems to distinguish the work of deaf adults from that of deaf classroom assistants, is not clear. Perhaps the distinction respondents were making lay in defining the cultural needs of the child, not just the academic needs, and hence in the prioritizing of a deaf person as role model rather than just a linguistic or academic resource. This subject clearly requires further investigation.

Employment patterns

The 36 projects reported the employment of 100 deaf people (Table 1.2). Of these, 42 were described as working full time, 51 as part time and 7 were volunteers – typically only paid expenses rather than a fee for the work they did. Reliable information about the exact number of hours the 'part-time' staff worked is not available, but what was important and perhaps surprising about this part-time group is that 43% ($n = 22$) of them were described as having 'permanent contracts' with the project. That is to say, they were not sessional or casual staff but played a substantial and consistent role. Of the full-time deaf employees, 86% ($n = 36$) had permanent contracts. In other words, well over half of the deaf staff working on the projects had secure employment, a finding that points to many of these projects being ones in which there was committed investment of time and resources and a professionalization of the service provided. These are not projects run by volunteers on an ad hoc basis.

However, this impression of well-established rather than ad hoc projects is somewhat contradicted by the finding that over half of the projects

Table 1.2 Number of deaf staff employed in the 35 projects

Number of (deaf) staff	Proportion of projects
1	18 (51%)
2–5	11 (31%)
6–10	5 (14%)
Over 10	1 (3%)

employed only one member of staff (only 14 of whom worked full time).

The likely professional isolation of people working in these single-person projects is further reinforced by the finding that one-third of these 18 projects reported having no contact whatsoever with similar projects in the UK and the remaining two-thirds only had 'occasional contact'. Given the extensive similarities in aims and underpinning philosophy of the projects, this lack of contact points to a failure to make the most of other projects' experience and expertise, missed opportunities for joint training and the pooling of resources, and a lack of a supportive network for deaf employees essentially fulfilling similar roles.

It should be remembered, however, that in contrast to this picture of small-scale isolated work are the 6 projects employing over 6 deaf staff. They accounted for 42% of all deaf employees working in the total sample of 36 projects. Not surprisingly, within these well-established teams, deaf staff occupied supervisory and senior roles, there were typically well-established training structures, routes to gaining professional qualifications in cases where staff began employment without them, and well-developed links with similar services to whom these projects often played a mentoring or advisory role. Although it is true to say that most of the projects displaying these characteristics had been established for a long time, these developments and structures were not automatic consequences of the longevity of projects. It was attention to training, qualification and professional development that were of significance.

Training, qualifications and professional development

Of the 100 employees associated with the 36 projects, 45 were described as possessing formal qualifications/professional accreditation and around half of these were employed in two of the largest projects described above. The finding that the majority of staff had no formal professional qualifications was not unexpected within the UK context, where very few deaf people have been enabled to access further or higher education, where there is not a large pool of professional trained deaf people, and many working in statutory services do so at unqualified grades (Young, Ackerman and Kyle, 1998).

The more pertinent issue in relation to these projects was what the training needs and training support structures were for deaf people once employed. Although 'being deaf' was a necessary and vital condition to fulfilling the roles these projects promoted, it was clearly not a sufficient condition in what could be highly complex and sensitive work with children and families. Information on identified training needs was supplied by 29 out of the 36 projects. These needs fell into three broad categories.

- **Child-related training.** This encompassed child development, skills in dealing with challenging behaviour, general skills in handling children and approaches to working with families as a whole. Of concern is that only three projects mentioned the need for any training in respect to child protection issues. Given that deaf employees are working directly with children and may be doing so alone and in the home, the failure to mention child protection training was worrying.
- **Gaining recognized professional qualifications.** There was a strong feeling, particularly from the larger projects, that although deaf staff may typically enter the work without qualifications, they should be provided with a means of gaining qualifications that are formally recognized, be it in teaching, social work, BSL/language instruction, or in specially tailored courses such as that for 'deaf instructors'. Once again it is the projects that are well-established over time, have secure and continued funding and a team of project workers who are likely to be in a better position to plan for such attainment amongst their staff.
- **Professional skills.** These included assertiveness and confidence building, becoming more aware of organizational structures and the wider service context and skills for working in partnership with families. 'Hearing awareness', particularly in relation to typical psychological reactions or emotional responses to having a deaf child, was also picked out.

Finally, it should be noted that the majority of respondents filling in the survey were hearing managers rather than the deaf employees themselves, and it was not possible to gauge the amount of consultation that had taken place over answers to this part of the survey. Deaf employees themselves could well have prioritized different training needs if the research had taken place through 'live' means of data collection such as interviews directly with them in BSL. It is an area of investigation that would warrant more attention.

Evaluation of impact

Given the rapid growth of these kinds of projects, issues in transition from short-term funding to established service and the more widespread development of an evidence-based service culture in the UK, the issue of whether and how projects had been evaluated was a key question. In 23 out of the 36 projects no evaluation had ever been carried out. In the rest, the most common form of evaluation was a simple user satisfaction survey in which families were asked for feedback, or less formally, any unsolicited comments are recorded. The following were typical descriptions of this approach to evaluation:

We evaluate each visit by taking parental comments, Teacher of the Deaf feedback and observed benefits. No overall evaluation though – more anecdotal.

We use questionnaires for parents/children to complete, regarding their views of services. We have regular meetings with families.

We have not established evaluation procedures but keep a file of comments and compliments.

The problem with this kind of evaluation is that, although it might pick up specific problems or dislikes from the service user perspective, any positive ratings of satisfaction tell us little. Satisfaction ratings are only as good as the level of pre-existing expectations a respondent might have, and are dependent on their wider knowledge of the range of alternative possibilities and outcomes. Essentially, if you do not expect much and have nothing to compare it with, satisfaction is always going to be high.

A few projects had completed evaluations as a requirement of continued funding. These were more like audits of how many families had received the service, what it had cost and so forth. Any measure of actual impact on child and family was not integral to such evaluations. Only two projects had sought independent evaluations, in both cases from university departments. One was undertaken some time ago and another was in progress.

In short, the impact of these projects is not well evaluated and the evidence base for their contribution to deaf child and family development is not well established. What is needed is a common instrument that all similar projects can use to collect data. The results from a large number of similar projects, although existing separately, if combined would enable a large enough sample for conclusions to be valid. On the other hand, too many local variables in service delivery may mean such an approach is not viable. A meta-analysis of all published evaluations worldwide of this kind of deaf adult intervention project is currently under way (Young, Clibbens and Sutherland, forthcoming) and will hopefully assist in the development of more usable evaluation tools on a local basis as well.

Conclusion

This study has demonstrated how intervention projects firmly underpinned by the significance of the 'deaf role' in working with families are on the increase, successfully attract both statutory and non-statutory funding and have the potential to exist as established parts of service provision for families. However, the limited size of many projects, their relative isolation from each other and lack of rigorous evaluation are all missed opportunities for the further development and strengthening of this approach to working with families.

Although this study was able to examine some trends over time, it was essentially a snapshot of current provision. Projects may now have been profiled, but there is no sense of their life history. Questions such as what challenges are faced at different points in the evolution of services and how these are met, remain unanswered. Similarly day-to-day operational concerns over such issues as referral patterns, inter-agency working and relationships between deaf and hearing staff have not been examined. Yet these issues are vital to understanding project development, staff support and impact.

All project staff and their line managers were invited to a follow-up one-day conference funded by the study. This provided a means of disseminating the findings but also of enabling projects to network with each other, gain support, and share experiences, materials and professional know how. Whether and how such a network could be sustained in the future remains to be seen, but clearly family projects underpinned by the linguistic and cultural interventions engendered in 'deaf roles' are firmly a part of the current landscape.

A more long-term question, perhaps, lies in how such projects may change as more and more deaf people take on professional occupations such as teachers of the deaf, social workers, nursery nurses and so forth. This will bring parents into increasingly routine contact with deaf people outside of a specially created 'deaf role model' framework for intervention. Will this eventually result in a reduced need for the projects we have studied – or will it mean that they become even more clearly defined in contrast to other experiences of deaf contact parents may have? The emerging pattern will be an interesting one to watch in the future.

Acknowledgements

The original research on which this chapter was based was funded by the Royal National Institute for Deaf People. We offer our sincere thanks to the many individual and services who responded to our surveys.

Chapter 2
Interaction with a deaf child: the contributions made by mother, father and sister

MEG SHEPHERD AND CLARE GALLAWAY

Background

Early identification of hearing loss and early intervention have focused professional minds on interaction in the primary learning environment of the home. In this chapter, we will look at the very particular challenges faced by the 90% of deaf children born into hearing families and negotiating an oral environment.

In this small-scale study, patterns of interaction between a hearing-impaired toddler and hearing family members were investigated. Its aim was to move beyond the traditional mother–child dyad to examine situations in which the child has to share the attention of a parent with a brother or sister, which is a more typical language-learning environment. The original study set out, firstly, to compare mother–child interaction with paternal and sibling styles. Secondly, it aimed at comparing and contrasting patterns of interaction in conversations where three family members were present (the triadic condition) with those in conversations between only two family members (the dyadic condition).

The data is taken from a set of recordings of conversations in a family consisting of mother, father, a deaf child (J) aged 2;6 and his hearing sister aged 4;9. Triadic conversations were between a parent, the deaf child and his sister (parent–child–child). Dyadic conversations were between a parent and the deaf child or his sister; and the conversations between the siblings (parent–J; parent–sister; J–sister).

Mapping interaction: a review of the literature

For a general view of the characteristics of conversational interaction with infants, we turn first to the literature on hearing children. The primary focus has been on the mother–child pair; fewer analyses have been made of father or sibling, and less attention still has been given to triadic and polyadic settings.

Mother–child interaction

Literature on conversational interaction between mothers and their young children suggests that the mother, tuned to the communicative competence of her child, is able to support and structure the infant's role in the conversation, providing early experience of turn-taking and topic maintenance (Snow, 1989; Barton and Tomasello, 1994; Davidson and Snow, 1996).

Father–child interaction

A number of common themes on maternal and paternal conversational differences have emerged since Gleason (1975) first proposed the 'bridge hypothesis'. This suggests that the secondary-caregiver father is less aware of the child's language and communicative abilities and is therefore a less supportive and more demanding conversational partner.

The following divergences from maternal style are described in the literature:

- paternal language is marked by a broader lexical range and contains more unusual vocabulary items
- utterances are shorter
- requests for clarification, wh-type questions and repetitions are more frequent
- corrections of the child's speech are less frequent
- total number of words in the conversation are fewer (Masur and Gleason, 1980; Rondal, 1980; McLaughlin et al, 1983; Hladik and Edwards, 1984; Bernstein-Ratner, 1988).

Breakdowns in communication occur more often with the father, who is also more likely to fail to acknowledge a child's attempt at communication than the mother (Tomasello, Conti-Ramsden and Ewert, 1990). Davidson and Snow (1996) found in contrast that the mothers in their study were the more challenging partners. Their language was more complex. They were more talkative and initiated more topics than fathers. In their ecological analysis of parent–infant relationships, Braungart-Rieker, Courtney and Garwood (1999) remind us that maternal/paternal differences transcend these tight pragmatic and linguistic parameters. Family functioning is shaped by a complex network of interconnecting influences that include parent and child characteristics but also incorporate social, economic and gender factors. Certain aspects of family type (single earner, dual earner; sex of child; parent sensitivity; state of marriage; infant emotionality) may differentially shape the father–infant/mother–infant relationship.

Paternal and maternal differences may run deep, but a number of authors have suggested that fathers' less contingent, more directive style may have developmental benefits for the child. McLaughlin et al (1983) refer to a 'differential experience' model, hypothesizing that the father's reduced sensitivity to the child's linguistic needs creates greater demands on the child and raises performance. In their examination of parental responsiveness, Tomasello, Conti-Ramsden and Ewert (1990) looked at the incidence of breakdowns in communication in the conversations of mothers and fathers with their young children (1;3 and 1;9). Conversational impasse was more likely with secondary-caregiver fathers. Not only did fathers ask children to clarify more frequently, but these requests did not usually make the breakdown element clear, placing the burden on the child. The implication drawn by the authors was that a less flexible partner will force the child to maximize his skills.

Harrison, Magill-Evans and Sadoway (2001) stress that instruments for measuring interaction need to recognize distinct father/mother styles. They used the Nursing Child Assessment Teaching Scale (NCATS) to measure fathers' play and involvement with their children under 3 and found they scored lower on a number of items – including sensitivity to cues and contingency – than the mothers on whom the scale was normed. The authors argue that difference should not be seen as deficiency, and lower cut-off scores may need to be used with fathers to avoid overestimating the number in need of intervention. The element of challenge in paternal styles needs to be retained to foster child growth.

Sibling interaction

Inflexibility is the hallmark of many of the sibling interactions studied. Sibling–infant conversations are shorter, with more non-verbal turns than mother–infant exchanges (Dunn and Kendrick, 1982; Vandell and Wilson, 1987). Children interacting with other children will apply simplified versions of the techniques for maintaining conversations learned with their mothers (Martinez, 1987). Sibling speech contains fewer questions and is more directive. Siblings are less likely to repair conversations when they break down than mothers (Mannle, Barton and Tomasello, 1991). As with fathers, non-acknowledgements are frequent (Tomasello and Mannle, 1985; Mannle, Barton and Tomasello, 1991).

Tomasello and Mannle (1985) showed that siblings' direct utterances to infants were fewer than mothers'. Their speech contained more direc-tives and fewer interrogatives. Siblings tended not to follow the infants' attentional focus. There were fewer interactions overall between infants and siblings. The conversations with siblings were shorter, and these end-stopped conversations were largely the effect of sibling non-acknowledgment and failure to take up and extend infant contributions.

Mannle, Barton and Tomasello (1991) compared their 16 subjects (22–26 months old) in two dyadic conditions – one with mother, the other with sibling (3;7–6;4). The authors' expectations were that sib-ling–infant conversations would be shorter, dominated by the sibling, and lack the cohesion of mother–infant exchanges. Mother–infant dyads were indeed found to have more conversations than sibling–infant dyads. Conversations were twice as long as child–child. The length of infants' turns and utterances remained constant across contexts, but they had more turns and spoke more often with mothers. Siblings often ignored infant utterances.

Along the lines of the father-bridge hypothesis, Tomasello and Mannle (1985) and Mannle, Barton and Tomasello (1991) formulated the sibling-bridge theory. Sibling unresponsiveness would make younger children more likely to adapt and persist when their message seems not to have been understood. Sibling inflexibility would prepare younger children for 'real-world' interaction with their peers.

Triadic interaction

In common with many of the studies of father and sibling styles, the lit-erature tends to present triadic interaction as a compromised environment for language learning, when contrasted with the dyad. In other words, when there are three people involved in the conversation, it is less likely to be helpful to the language learning child. Interactions involving an adult and two or more children, it suggests, will be marked by reduced adult responsiveness. The adult in Schaffer and Liddell (1984) broke down the interplay into a series of dyads rather than developing a truly polyadic style. Woollett (1986) found that the major-ity of maternal utterances in triads were addressed to the older child. In contrast, Pappas Jones and Adamson's (1987) mothers addressed the majority of utterances to the younger child. However, when two chil-dren were present, mothers used more directive language. Miller, Vollig and McElwain (2000) looked at the triad as a means of socialization rather than a locus for language learning. Their analysis of jealousy reac-tions, when parents interacting with a toddler and pre-school-age sibling were asked to focus on just one of the children, revealed differ-ences in the way parents regulated the resulting behaviours. Fathers behaved similarly regardless of the age of the sibling. This less contin-gent, less adaptive approach lends support to the role of the father as a more challenging partner.

Woollett's (1986) study saw the tentative emergence of a new theme, suggesting possible advantages to triadic interaction. Although conversations involving three participants were found to be less sensitive to the needs of the youngest child, they also provide a more stimulating and challenging environment. However, this enrichment might not be available to the younger child, who is less directly involved than mother or sibling.

The theme of triads providing language and learning opportunities was recently explored by Strapp (1999) who looked at how young children's syntactic development might proceed through negative evidence in different family configurations (dyadic, triadic and tetradic). Her subjects were 14 children (2;3) and their siblings (4;1). She found that it was not how many were involved in the interaction that correlated with level of feedback but who was involved: there was reduced feedback in sibling-involved triads. Although for just under half the children the mother-dyad was the primary source of feedback, for 21% this was the father–child dyad and, for some triads, and tetrads served this function.

Triadic interaction – the sibling effect reconsidered

Barton and colleagues have also reviewed the contribution of siblings within a triadic setting. Barton and Tomasello (1991) suggest a possible advantage to sibling-involved triads, noting that triads have their own dynamic. In interactions involving 19- and 24-month olds, their mothers and pre-school siblings (3–5 years), they found the following features:

- children as young as 19 months were involved in triadic interaction
- triadic interaction was 3 times longer than dyadic interaction
- infants and siblings were more likely to join in or continue a conversation than initiate one.

Barton and Strosberg (1997) revisited the triad theme, but this time with mother–twin–twin (mean age 2;3). They found parallels between these and the 1991 triads, suggesting that these behaviours are an effect of the triad and reiterating the potential benefits of contexts with more than one child. Triadic contexts can move conversational skills on rather than retarding them, and may give later-borns a pragmatic advantage, since they have daily opportunities to practise the early conversational skills of joining into a conversation appropriately and negotiating turn-taking with more than one person.

Tremblay-Leveau, Leclerc and Nadel (1999), comparing the communication skills of 16- and 23-month old twins and singletons in triads, confirmed a triadic advantage for the twins. They propose that assessment of twins' language skills within a dyadic context underestimates their abilities. In the more familiar triadic setting, they are able to show their skill in verbally and pragmatically managing a multi-speaker conversation.

The literature on hearing children shows

- differences in the way mothers and fathers talk to their infants and toddlers
- the impact the presence of two children can have on an adult's style of interaction, making it less contingent.

In contrast to the latter finding, however, two studies (Barton and Tomasello, 1991; Barton and Strosberg, 1997) have suggested that inter-action between an adult and two children can advance the children's conversational skills by providing them with

- experience of longer conversations
- more opportunities for joining in an established conversation
- practice in shifting attention between two conversational partners.

Interaction between deaf children and their parents

Access to language, signed and spoken, can be a problem for deaf children in hearing families. Harris (2000) outlines the difficulties faced by hearing mothers in managing the attention of their children and meeting the demands of a visual language. Contingent responding, techniques for making sign available, and the incremental adaptation of language input to reflect the child's growing linguistic maturity may be problematic in hearing mother–deaf child dyads. Synchrony and reciprocity, the hallmarks of effective interaction, may not emerge without support (e.g. through deaf role models or the explicit teaching of communication strategies) (Vaccari and Marschark, 1997).

Three recent articles have looked at the patterns of influence of parental hearing status on deaf children's play and attention skills in the early years.

Spencer and Meadow-Orlans (1996) examined the impact of the child's language level and maternal responsiveness on children's play. Their 43 dyads, studied when the children were 9, 12 and 18 months, were distributed across the following groups: h(earing) child–H(earing) parent, d(eaf) child–D(eaf) parent, d(eaf) child–H(earing) parent. At 12 months, they found no main effect for language in the emergence of symbolic play. At both 12 and 18 months, however, more developed language was linked with a higher level of symbolic play.

By 18 months, the strongest correlation with highest level play was maternal responsiveness. Parental contingency scaffolds child skill. Non-contingent responding in mismatched hearing-status dyads has implications for skill development. At 12 months, both groups of deaf children were producing less representational play than hearing children. By 18 months, dH children's symbolic play was least complex, but dD children were producing the same amount of pre-planned symbolic play (the highest category of play) as hearing children. The authors suggest that both deaf groups show similar levels of play at 12 months in the solitary and collaborative conditions, because maternal presence is not supporting the more advanced skill. Maternal verbal commentary (which scaffolds play to a higher level) is inaccessible (at least partially) to the deaf child of a hearing mother. Deaf mothers of younger deaf children produce fewer signs, which would have a similar effect in reducing verbal support to the child. By 18 months, however, the dD children have 'caught up' with the hearing children, following a different route to the higher skill level. Significantly, dH children continue to lag, spending much less time at the highest level of play.

The challenge for early intervention is to learn from deaf families and to encourage hearing parents to incorporate techniques for supporting deaf children's play development.

Prezbindowski, Adamson and Lederberg (1998) looked at 48 20–24 month olds, divided equally into hearing child–hearing mother dyads and deaf child–hearing mother dyads. Their interest was in the coordination of attention between people, objects and symbols. They found that time spent in joint attention increases during the second year for all children, but that joint attention was qualitatively different for deaf children. At the end of the second year, deaf children's primary type was coordinated joint attention, but for hearing children joint attention was 'symbol-infused' (that is the joint object of interest was symbolic – words, symbolic play, symbolic gestures – not concrete). Joint attention follows a similar path in the first 18 months for deaf and hearing children. In the second half of the second year, however, when context is less used by hearing children, a pattern of divergence emerges. The authors propose that intervention programmes teach hearing parents to coordinate the more extensive episodes of joint attention in the second year with the introduction of symbolic play and language. Their proposal was that deaf children need to be visually primed for symbolic communication to be effective.

Bornstein et al (1999) studied 89 children in a four-group design: h/H; h/D; d/H; d/D. Their aim was to re-examine the nature of the links between symbolic language and play, by posing two questions:

- Do language and play manifest a common underlying semiotic function?
- Do they spring from the same semiotic source in early development but diverge later on?

Where dyads were mismatched, solitary symbolic play and collaborative symbolic play initiated by the child were correlated with measures of expressive and receptive language. This was not the case with matched dyads. However, when symbol play was initiated by the adult partner, which produces a more advanced level of play, language and play did not covary. Covariance, the authors argue, is the mark of an early stage of development. The covariance of language and play at later stages will only be seen when one system is damaged. When symbolic play is supported and structured by a more competent partner, the higher level, uncorrelated state will be achieved. Though initially aspects of a common underlying symbolic capacity in early language and play, the two symbol systems differentiate in later development. The authors' message is an optimistic one, suggesting that compromise to one symbol system does not necessarily impinge on the other. One can work to the dyad's strengths, using the child's skill in one area as a platform for improving the less developed representational ability.

The triadic context: conversational interaction in families with a deaf child

To our knowledge, no research has been carried out to date on the relative contributions of parents and siblings in dyadic and triadic conversations when one of the infants is deaf. As we mentioned earlier, conversational interaction within families will frequently involve more than two participants. Consideration of the features of triadic conversational interaction, therefore, is important when we are trying to understand the circumstances of language acquisition and in particular, the development of conversational skills.

Research themes

In comparing our family with a deaf child with the research findings on hearing families, we were guided by the following questions.

- Would hearing-status mismatch compromise the sensitivity of mother to her son, and make her as challenging a conversational partner as father and sibling?
- Would the findings of Barton and Tomasello (1991) and Barton and Strosberg (1997) be reflected in our conversations involving 3 people, i.e.
  - would there be longer conversations between 3 people?
  - would the younger (deaf) child join into these conversations?
  - would he be able to shift his attention between and keep the attention of two conversational partners?

In order to look at some of the themes from the literature on hearing children, conversations within a family with a deaf child were recorded and analysed.

Data

J was 2;6 at the time of the study; his sister, 4;9. J had a severe hearing loss and had been bilaterally aided for one year. At the time of the study, his vocalizing was marked by consonant and vowel variety and the emergence of some recognizable words and learned phrases.

The family were recorded once a week over a period of 4 weeks. Sessions lasted 1 hour, of which approximately 30 minutes were taped. Each session recorded play between one parent and the two children. Two sessions feature the father and two the mother. Transcripts were made of the middle 10 minutes of each recorded half hour.

Analysis of data

Data analysis was aimed at conveying the shape of conversational interaction and the role played by the parents, and by the hearing and deaf siblings in the interchange.

Conversational boundaries

The unit of structural analysis was the conversation. This was defined thematically as a sequence of utterances between speakers on a common topic of interest (see Mannle, Barton and Tomasello, 1991). Conversational boundaries were determined thus: the conversation was deemed to have ended when a new topic of interest was introduced or when one partner had to break away to caretake or chastise one of the children.

If one partner moved away, but the other two partners stayed with the topic under discussion, the conversation was judged to continue. Non-verbal involvement in the conversation was assessed on the following criteria: interest in the topic under discussion, evinced by physical proximity, gaze, touch or use of objects (Spencer, 1993). Inter-rater reliability for conversational boundaries was 85%; disagreements were resolved by discussion.

Measures of language and conversation analysis

A number of quantitative measures were carried out, in order to characterize these conversations and to provide a basis for comparing them with the studies of hearing children mentioned above (Table 2.1).

Did the other members of the family modify their speech to J?

There was plenty of evidence that all members of the family modified their language when talking to J. They all used shorter utterances when

Table 2.1 Language and conversation analysis

Measure	What it reveals
Mean length of utterance Length of longest utterance	Sensitivity to the listening and language needs of the deaf child
Utterance totals Word totals	Participant's talkativeness
Number of turns addressed by each participant to each of the others in the conversation	Whose attention different family members were most likely to be soliciting
Initiations and terminations in each conversation	Who was taking control of the conversation
Ratio of turns	Who was taking most turns in the conversation

talking to him, particularly in dyadic conversations. There were also differences in the 'density' of language addressed to him. Father was most wordy and sister the least. In triadic conversations, J was the linguistic focus, with the majority of parental utterances addressed to him.

Were there differences between mother and father?

Mother and father structured the interaction in different ways, with mother segmenting her involvement with the children into dyadic episodes. In other words, she tended to break up the conversation and address one child at a time rather then both at once. Conversational control (in terms of who initiated and who ended conversations) was largely exercised by the parents, with sister taking some responsibility, but J very little.

Although the average length of conversations with both mother and father was very similar, there were some interesting differences, seen primarily in the ways they dealt with the pressure of interacting with two children. Father combined his own and the siblings' contributions into extended triadic sequences. Mother focused sequentially on one or other of the children.

Comparison of this study with Barton and Tomasello (1991) and Barton and Strosberg (1997)

To compare the three-way conversations within our family with those of the hearing families in the published studies (Table 2.2), we looked at

- the relative distribution of conversations involving two and three people

- the length of the two types of conversation
- the role of the sibling
- evidence of the younger child's ability to break into a conversation.

Table 2.2 Percentage of conversations that involve two or three people

	Present study		Barton and Tomasello (1991)	
	Dyadic	Triadic	Dyadic	Triadic
Session 1 (F)	20	80	77	23
Session 2 (M)	72	28		
Session 3 (F)	27	73		
Session 4 (M)	75	25		

F, father involved; M, mother involved.

Barton and Tomasello found that, even when three people were present, the majority of conversations involved only two of them. Sessions where the mother is involved are close to the Barton and Tomasello data: with father, however, there is a strong triadic bias, providing further evidence of parents' different approaches to managing the conversational demands of two children.

Length of conversations

Father's exchanges with the toddler and his sibling accord well with the published data (Table 2.3). Mother's conversations with J alone, however, are longer than both mother–toddler–sibling and mother–sibling conversations. The mother's style places a premium on focused dyadic interaction with the hearing-impaired child, whereas the father favours triadic over dyadic interaction.

Table 2.3 Comparison of average lengths of conversations involving two and three people (in turns)

	Father–toddler–sibling	Father–sibling	Father–toddler
Session 1	29	6	0
Session 3	25	6	5

	Mother–toddler–sibling	Mother–sibling	Mother–toddler
Session 2	26	4	42
Session 4	14	15	25

Barton and Tomasello (1991)	Mother–infant–sibling (3 times longer than mother–infant or mother-sibling)
Barton and Strosberg (1997)	Mother–twin–twin (5 times longer than mother–twin)

Role of the sibling

There is little direct contact between siblings in our study or in those of
Barton and colleagues (Table 2.4). In our family, there is more sibling
interaction when the parent is present and able to set up situations that
facilitate contact between the children.

Table 2.4 Comparison of number of turns addressed to toddler by sibling and
parent

	Session 1 (F)		Session 2 (M)		Session 3 (F)		Session 4 (M)	
	Triadic	Dyadic	Triadic	Dyadic	Triadic	Dyadic	Triadic	Dyadic
Sister to J	14	0	7	8	6	0	1	0
Parent to J	52	0	9	22	53	3	8	47

Barton and Tomasello (1991)	Sibling–infant conversations rare at both 19 and 24 months
Barton and Strosberg (1997)	No twin A–twin B conversations

The deaf child's contribution to the conversation

In the studies by Barton and colleagues, two-thirds of the children's first
turns joined into or continued a conversation; that is, they were active
contributors to the conversation. Our impression was that J was a more
passive partner. His contributions were often in the form of comments
meant only for himself (Table 2.5). Without a specific addressee, these
comments would not move the conversation on, unless they were taken
up and developed by a more competent partner. Their status might thus
be compared to a very young child's non-intentional vocalization which
a parent interprets as meaningful. J's comments are not conversational-
ly significant in themselves but are tailored by his partners into the
ongoing conversation.

Table 2.5 Number of toddler J's turns which have no specific addressee

	Session 1 (F)	Session 2 (M)	Session 3 (F)	Session 4 (M)
Total turns	87	68	77	49
Undirected turns	46	37	51	17

Father replies to J's undirected turns and uses them to loop sister
back into the conversation, keeping the three-way conversation going.
Mother uses the ambiguity of addressee to create additional opportunities for dyadic interaction with J.

Interaction in mismatched hearing-status triads

Unlike the children in the studies by Barton and colleagues, J has conversations built around him. However, in common with these children, for whom only 11–19% of turns were initiating a topic, J makes very few initiations. This contrasts with older deaf children and their use of initiation as a means of controlling the conversation (Wood et al, 1986).

It would be interesting to study how initiations develop in deaf and hearing children in the early years and to compare development in deaf and hearing families. The hypothesis would be that in an optimally functioning environment, deaf children would not have to develop initiation as an adaptive strategy. Would this be borne out by the use made of it by deaf children in deaf families?

No follow-up study was undertaken to track J.'s development of joining-in strategies in triadic environments. The children who were joining in and continuing conversations in Barton and Tomasello (1991) and Barton and Strosberg (1997) were 19–24 months and 2;3 respectively. Did J begin to do this at his corrected hearing age (which is a year behind his chronological age), or was there further delay, compounded by his reduced access to acoustic cues and less well-developed vocabulary?

Barton and Tomasello's 19-month-olds were involved in triadic joint-attentional episodes, but, as the authors point out, this is the earliest age at which this more complex form of attention sharing (as opposed to the infant–partner–object mode) has been found and the skill continued to develop in their subjects between 19 and 24 months. The supported triadic attention which characterizes many of our deaf child's interactions might represent a scaffolding stage of an emerging skill. Further studies of hearing and deaf children in the second year of life might show whether this scaffolded stage is a recurrent feature. It might also be instructive to follow the development of triadic attention from about 9 to 19 months in hearing and deaf children and track the shift from object to person as the third point of the communication triangle.

Summary

By splitting her attention between the children and breaking the interplay down into a series of dialogues, the mother simplifies the interactional environment.

The father seems a more challenging partner. His wordiness and occasionally very long utterances to J provide a linguistic challenge of that is not present in mother's less dense and more compact speech. He also exploits the triadic situation, building more three-cornered interactions.

Maternal and paternal styles are complementary, with the father providing a transition to the difficulties of multi-speaker environments, whereas the mother continues to provide highly structured support for J.'s growing conversational skills.

His sister's limited engagement with J lends some support to the 'sibling-bridge' hypothesis. Is there also evidence of 'sibling-benefit' in the form of a more stimulating language environment? Although there is little direct verbal contact between brother and sister, she does provide a store of imaginative language in the monologues with which she accompanies her play and models the pragmatics of 'breaking into' and continuing an ongoing conversation.

The study reported here was small-scale and focused on a deaf child in a hearing family. Further work is essential to extend our knowledge of the experience of deaf children communicating in triadic contexts. This would need to map the coordinates of interaction in a variety of settings (deaf children in deaf and hearing families; hearing children in hearing and deaf families). Studies would have to be longitudinal, tracing the development of the young child's role in triadic interaction over time.

A more secure knowledge base might then allow intervention to optimize triadic interaction in hearing families with deaf children and complement the current focus on dyadic interaction.

Chapter 3
Conversations with young deaf children in families where English is an additional language

MERLE MAHON

This chapter is about communication between deaf children and their family members in homes where English is an additional language (EAL). It is based on a recent study in which Conversation Analysis (CA) methods were used to examine conversations between 7-year-old deaf children from Sylheti-speaking families and their family members. The analysis yielded preliminary and productive insights. Similar data from hearing EAL children and from English-speaking deaf children are included for comparison.

The main research question was: Are there any outstanding features of talk with deaf EAL children that could shed light on the way such children acquire the linguistic skills needed for conversation? This is based on the premise that conversation between children and mature speakers (parents, older siblings) is the main avenue for development of the child's home language (Snow, 1995; Chiat, 2000). One of the features of conversations between adults and children is the question and answer sequence, well documented for deaf and hearing children (Gallaway and Richards, 1994). Here, such sequences of talk with deaf EAL children will be explored.

Key terms: an explanation

The words 'deaf' and 'deafness' (BDA, 1996) are used here to mean the range of permanent, prelingual sensori-neural hearing impairments (as distinct from conductive or central impairments) which are of sufficient severity to lead to problems in communication using spoken language. This use of the term 'deaf' is not to be confused with the term 'Deaf' which is currently used in the UK when referring to the Deaf community and culture whose mode of communication is sign, and for whom British Sign Language (BSL) is their first and home language. None of the families taking part in the research considered their children to be 'Deaf'.

The acronym EAL (English as an additional language) is used to characterize individuals and families who use several languages and/or dialects including English. The focus on English here is not to detract from the families' rich language repertoire, but to highlight complex issues concerning English for deaf EAL children growing up in the UK. The research referred to in this chapter was conducted in the East End of London, with families from the Bangladeshi-British community. The home language of the families who took part in the research is Sylheti, a language closely related to Bengali, spoken in the northern Bangladeshi province of Sylhet (Chalmers, 1996). Family members are also skilled in other languages – standard Bengali, Arabic, and other Asian languages, such as Hindi, or Punjabi. In addition, they use English: one or both parents may have studied English as a foreign language (in the UK or elsewhere), and older siblings at school in the UK used a variety of forms of English depending on their level of proficiency. Sylheti-speaking Bangladeshi-British people are a significantly numerous EAL group in the UK (Office of National Statistics, 2001). Schools in London's East End have many students from EAL families presenting a unique challenge to teachers and other professionals such as speech and language therapists and psychologists (Storkey, 1994; Turner, 1996; RCSLT, 1998; Winter, 1998; Baker and Eversley, 2000). Furthermore, recent studies indicate that there are significant numbers of deaf children from Asian families (Vanniasegaram, Tungland and Bellman, 1993; Naeem and Newton, 1996; Sutton and Rowe, 1997).

The particular meaning of the word 'conversation' used here requires explanation. Conversation requires that the participants are partners in the exercise, who take turns to speak (or to sign) and to listen (or watch) in a relatively orderly manner, doing so using words (or signs) in a way that is coherent and accessible to each other, in order to achieve mutual understanding. If this is not achieved, conversation requires that one participant will indicate her/his difficulty to the other, making it possible for that difficulty to be resolved. The participants indicate to each other that they have understood each other's meanings by the way in which they design their turns. It is taken for granted that they will be using the same language. As will be seen later, this is not the case in some of the data that will be discussed. An underlying assumption is that the participants are competent in the skills required for the task, which are, simply put, speaking (or signing), listening (or watching) and using the appropriate social and cultural conventions of interaction.

A useful method for studying conversation

The choice of method for the study was motivated by the need to account for the way in which the children and the adults manage their communication so that they demonstrably achieve mutual understanding. After careful consideration of various methodologies used in the analysis of discourse and of spoken interactions, Conversation Analysis (CA) was deemed to be the most appropriate method (Hutchby and Wooffitt, 1998). The reason for this is that the inductive, data-driven premise of CA, arising from ethnomethodology, enables the analyst to examine 'talk-in-interaction' between two or more participants, in detail, without resorting to intuitive assumptions, or applying preconceived categories. This differs from traditional linguistic analyses which draw on analytic methods from functional linguistics (e.g. Fairclough, 1992). In CA, descriptions of interactional behaviours (such as utterances, non-verbal behaviours, pauses) are made by using the same normative procedures for recognizing those behaviours as are used by the participants themselves. In this way, the design of each participant's behaviour (or 'turn' in the talk), and the sequential implications of that turn can be described and accounted for. Thus from the careful documentation of every aspect of each participant's contribution to the talk, the interactionally constructed meaning of the talk becomes accessible to the analyst.

The samples of conversation to be discussed were recorded in the homes of each of seven children who took part in the study: three 7-year-old deaf children (2 EAL and 1 English-speaking) (see end of chapter for audiological details about the deaf children); two 7-year-old hearing children (one EAL and one English-speaking) and two younger hearing children (one EAL and one English-speaking) whose language level more or less matched that of the deaf children. For this chapter, a selection of data samples taken from the activity of looking at photo albums or picture books with mother, father or older sister is discussed. These interactions are obviously not entirely 'naturally occurring' insofar as the interaction was set up by the researcher and was recorded. Nevertheless, the analyses provided a unique insight into the interaction which is relatively free from preconceived notions, leaving open the possibility of achieving new insights.

Why study the spoken conversations of deaf EAL children?

Firstly, seen in a broad perspective, conversation can be described as the

> primary medium of interaction in the social world and the medium through which children are socialised into the linguistic and social conventions of a society (Drew, 1990:1)

Secondly, it is in conversations that the well-documented difficulties of deaf children with speaking and listening are most apparent (Gallaway and Woll, 1994; Paul and Quigley, 2000). These are also skills which present difficulties in English conversation for learners of English who may have no problems in their home language. How are these language skills acquired? One aspect of this complex process will be discussed here.

Conversation between adults and children is a fundamental ingredient of language acquisition

The literature of child language research in the English-speaking world is packed with studies about the role of language input to, and language interaction with, normally hearing and developing children in a western (British), industrialized, monolingual (English) context (Chiat, 2000; Fletcher and MacWhinney, 1995). Essentially, conversations between adults and children are regarded as being one of the main avenues for the child's language development, so that a child's first language will be the family's home language and will be learned from mature speakers of that language in the home environment. It is assumed that the child, who is regarded as a conversational partner from a very early age, will be learning the same language as that spoken by the family. This language learning-teaching is a mutual accomplishment in which the mature speaker adopts a 'child-centred' style of talking to her/his child in order to promote language development, for example, s/he may modify the structure of her/his language to suit the perceived ability of the child to understand.

Cross-cultural and cross linguistic studies seem to indicate that most of the assumptions underlying the western 'child-centred' approach can be applied to conversations between adults and children in other languages and cultures (see Lieven, 1994 for a comprehensive review). Fernald and Morikawa (1993: 637) make the case for a culturally widespread 'infant-directed speech style' including features found in English, such as exaggerated prosody and frequent repetition, which is observable in many different languages, and which they suggest is manifested in response to 'universal characteristics and response tendencies of the human infant' Fernald and Morikawa (1993:654). However, other findings suggest that this view is too simplistic, since children learn to talk in a wide variety of cultural environments quite different from ours. A child-centred style may be helpful to western children, but it may not be essential for all children.

Cross-cultural studies however do not inform us about the situation of concern here, which is what happens in EAL families living in the UK. In other words, how does the language acquisition process proceed – is this child-centred approach one that is found when adults talk to their children in minority linguistic and cultural communities such as the Bangladeshi-British? There is no substantial body of information which directly concerns language development in EAL children per se. However, research in recent years has addressed related issues, particularly in the field of education (Gregory, 1996, 1998; Edwards, 1998; Blackledge, 2000) and special educational needs (Cline, 1998; Diniz, 1999). The work is encouraged by bodies such as the National

Association for Language Development in the Curriculum (NALDIC, 2001) which provides information and training for teachers. The requirements of the National Literacy Strategy (DfEE, 1998, 2001a) must be followed. Schools are supported in their work with EAL children by funding from the Ethnic Minority Achievement and Traveller Children Achievement Grant (DfEE, 2001b). There is also a growing body of knowledge about cultural issues to do with attitudes to health provision, disability and illness and the uptake of health related services (Ahmad, 1993; Shah, 1995; Ahmad and Atkin, 1996; Lau, 2000; Siraj-Blatchford and Clarke, 2000). Ahmad et al (1998) and Sharma and Love (1991) have written about deaf people from ethnic minority groups. Although all of this research contributes to our understanding to some extent, there is a substantial dearth of research concerning language development per se in deaf EAL children, and how fostering this development is similar to or different from that found with English-speaking deaf children and hearing EAL children. The following section addresses some of these issues.

The case for deaf EAL children

The child-centred approach to fostering language development discussed above is built on some underlying assumptions that may not be appropriate when considering deaf EAL children. The first assumption to question here is that of the first language. In many EAL families living in the UK, the first language is the home language. However this may not always be the case. When the parents taking part in the current research were asked the question, what is your deaf child's first language, the Bangladeshi-British parents replied 'English!' even though they had stated that their own (and their hearing children's) first language is Bengali (Sylheti). Why this was the case is interesting: it is likely that the families had been recommended by professionals to speak one language, English, to their deaf child. This is not unusual – in the UK, English is often recommended as the one language that should be used (Chamba, Ahmad and Jones, 1998), for reasons such as the benefit to the child's future education, which will be in the English medium.

There is also a generally held view that it is 'better' for deaf children to only be exposed to one language, but only a small amount of evidence to supports this view (Cunningham-Andersson and Andersson, 1999). There is a noticeable gap in the research literature here. Although there is research into sign bilingualism where there is evidence attesting to the benefits of deaf children learning signed and spoken languages at the same time (Petitto et al, 2001), there is simply no published research concerning deaf EAL children in this country which would inform us about the possible advantages or disadvantages of using home language with that child, and then allowing English to develop later on as an additional language.

From research with hearing EAL children, however, evidence abounds for the positive value of having two or more languages (Hoffmann, 1991; Romaine, 1994; de Houwer, 1995; Baker, 2000). Obviously, many factors have a bearing on an EAL child's language development, not the least being the time of the child's life at which the additional language is introduced. For hearing EAL children, English may be used at home by older siblings or heard on television, but the first real exposure could come when the child starts school. Children may then become somewhat separated from their home language because they have to master English in order to progress through our school system, and in effect they become 'emergent bilinguals' (Gregory, 1998).

This 'separation' from home language may occur very early for deaf children, especially if deafness is diagnosed relatively early. As soon as a diagnosis is made, rehabilitation procedures are set in place (NDCS, 1996). For example, deaf children can be given full-time nursery placements earlier than hearing children, so that they can be assessed fully in order to predict their educational needs (DfEE, 2000). A variety of health and education professionals, the vast majority of whom are English-speaking, will become involved with the deaf children at this early stage. They will all be concerned to foster the child's language development, and this means making a decision about which language should be used at home. It is at this point that a recommendation about only using English at home could be made. If one or other of the parents or other family members do not speak English, this strategy, albeit well-motivated, can cause huge difficulties for the communication between the deaf child and the family, as will be shown in the data samples for Kh and A later on. The intervention by professionals at an early age makes the EAL deaf child's experience of language learning very different indeed from that of either an English-speaking deaf child or a hearing EAL child. The findings in this study are informative here, giving some insight into the language experience at home. Much more research is needed, for example, to inform us about what happens at school, and how language development proceeds for deaf children and for hearing EAL children in both their home language and in English.

However, let us return to deaf children and their conversations. The following section will discuss some of the characteristics which research has shown can distinguish deaf children's conversations from that of hearing children.

Conversations with deaf children

Characterizing how conversations with deaf children differ from conversations with hearing children is not straightforward. Deaf children do not form an homogenous group, neither do the adults who are involved with them, thus making descriptions of 'typical' conversations difficult. Furthermore, many studies of deaf children's conversations are based on a traditional linguistic analysis of each participants' contributions to the conversation, and do not provide insight into how the participants go about actually constructing a mutually coherent conversation. Nevertheless, the indications from the research literature are that deaf children are less 'responsive' in conversation, and that adults talking to them tend to be 'controlling' (see Gallaway and Woll, 1994 for a comprehensive review; Lederberg and Everhart, 2000). By this is meant that the adults 'control' the interaction by modifying their input into 'restrictive' language, for example by frequent use of imperatives, very short sentences, the employment of a repetitive, narrow vocabulary and the use of questions (Gallaway, Hostler and Reeves, 1990; Musselman and Churchill, 1992, 1993). Controlled conversations are often heard in the classroom, 'teacher language', as the seminal work of Wood and his colleagues has demonstrated (Wood et al, 1986). However, as will be seen in the data discussed later, and as we know from common experience, when adults talk to children much 'teacher language' is used, no matter where the interaction is taking place. The frequency of occurrence of 'teacher language' and 'control' is often what differentiates talk between adults and deaf children from that between adults and hearing children. Lyon (1985) suggests that maternal control (using teacher language) in particular, could constitute 'a secondary and cumulative impediment' (p. 127) to language development in the deaf child. However, Gallaway and Woll (1994) indicate that this control could be also seen as an appropriate adjustment made by the mother or carer to language input as a result of their assessment of the child's receptive language levels. They add that restrictive language may well be appropriate for a 'still incompetent learner' (Gallaway and Woll (1994:202), thus giving a positive spin to the notion of 'control'. Thus features of controlled talk, such as question–answer sequences, can also be seen as a useful device for fostering the child's language development.

Question–answer sequences in a CA framework

In her analysis of parent–child interactions, Tarplee (1996) has shown that question–answer sequences can be seen to do important interactional work that facilitates language teaching and learning. She demonstrated that parents assisted in their children's acquisition of lexical and articulatory knowledge by engaging the children in labelling sequences where a 'test' question is asked by the adult (who knows the answer). Although Tarplee's work concerns very young hearing children, it is of relevance here, because the labelling, question–answer sequence is a frequent feature of conversations with deaf children of all ages.

To illustrate, some fragments of conversation are analysed below. This illustration will provide a useful prelude to understanding the data presented later. It will also show how the conversational turn structure in a question–answer sequence can be seen as benefiting language acquisition.

A key to the transcription notation is given at the end of the chapter.

In CA terms, the talk quoted below follows a typical pattern of three turns, in an orderly progression in which speakers take their allocated turn (Sacks, Schegloff and Jefferson, 1974). This progression indicates that the talk is 'locally managed' (Schegloff, 1992). Thus, the sequence is usually initiated by the adult (first turn), followed by the child's response (second turn), succeeded by the adult's receipt of (i.e. response to) the child's turn (third turn).

In the first two examples, fragments E1 and E2 (see Figs 3.1–3.3), E is a hearing 4-year-old EAL boy, talking to his 15-year-old sister, S. Their home language is Sylheti, in which both E and S are fluent. S has been at school in London for 6 years, and she also speaks good English. E is at nursery and is picking up some English there. In their conversation, S and E use both Sylheti and English. In the data fragments, words that were translated from Sylheti into colloquial English are printed in italics. Translation of talk from Sylheti into English was done by two independent translators working from the original tapes. For more details concerning these translations, and the transcriptions, see Mahon (1997).

In fragment E1, the typical three-turn structure described above is observed. S chooses to use a question structure in order to prompt E into a labelling answer. The analysis shows that her question is designed as a 'test' question, since it becomes clear that she knows the answer.

```
  1 S:    what is this ((points to picture of helicopter))
  2 E:    Helicopter
->3 S:    Yeah helicopter

         (1.0)
```

Figure 3.1 Fragment E1

Using a CA approach, it is possible to analyse this sequence of talk as follows:

- Line 1: S designs her sentence in this turn as a question. By doing this, she obliges E to give an answer in line 2.
- Line 2: E gives his candidate answer to the question.
- Line 3: S designs her turn here in such a way as to make it clear to E that she has understood his answer and that his answer was appropriate: her turn contains a direct lexical reference to the second turn, in which E has answered the question, (she repeats the word 'helicopter'). She also directly refers to E's turn in her prosody – her intonation on the word 'helicopter' mirrors his. For good measure, she also adds a confirmatory 'yeah'.

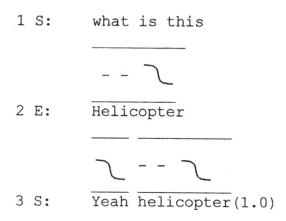

1 S: what is this

2 E: Helicopter

3 S: Yeah helicopter(1.0)

Figure 3.2 Fragment E1[A]

In fragment E1a (Figure 3.2), phonetic detail is added to the transcription to highlight these details (see Tarplee, 1996). E and S have understood each other perfectly here, and have displayed their understanding to each other. Using CA terminology, this sequence of talk can therefore be considered to have been locally managed (turns were taken sequentially in an orderly manner) and, the talk was 'interactionally managed' (Schegloff, 1992) since the two speakers have indicated clearly that they have understood each other's meanings. To put this in another way, 'intersubjectivity' between the speakers is shown to have been achieved.

The meaning of intersubjectivity requires further explanation here. Using the example of the sequence in fragment E1: by responding to the question (in the first turn) the answerer, E, manifests in his answer (in the second turn) a matrix of understandings of the prior question turn. These understandings include:

- that it is his turn to talk
- that the prior utterance has been understood as being a question
- that the grammar of that question was understood
- that the content of the question was understood.

Furthermore, having received the answer, the asker of the original question, S, then has the opportunity in the next turn to display her understanding of that answer (in the third turn) (Schegloff, 1992).

Hence, the design of the third turn (as a place in which lexical or phonetic checks are provided) is an important clue to whether or not there is local and interactional management of the talk, and to whether intersubjectivity is achieved.

What happens when there is a disagreement or a misunderstanding? As mentioned above, the third turn is an important locus for further interactional work to be done. It is used as a place where misunderstandings are acknowledged and if necessary, repair can be initiated, as can be seen in the next example (fragment E2) taken from the same conversation between E and his sister. Here not only does the question–answer sequence do the interactional work of 'teaching/learning' labels, but it also provides an opportunity to do repair work in which S is able to guide E in attaining an appropriate lexical label.

```
  1 S:      what uh kind of's this ((points to picture
            of the gun on the front of a fighter jet))
  2 E:      uh: (2.1) rocket
->3 S:      no: nearly=
  4 E:          uh
  5 S:      =wha are these these fighter planes innit (1.0)
            the war planes (1.2) they shoot people down=
```

```
  6 E:      =there front gun ((points to picture of gun on
                                          fighter jet))
```

```
  7 S:        gun
      (6.7)
```

Figure 3.3 Fragment E2

In line 3, S acknowledges E's answer to her first question in line 1. She does this by refuting E's answer, but also encouraging his attempt by saying 'no: nearly'. She does not allow him to take a turn (line 4) by overlapping his start 'uh', and she continues to ask another question which is designed to include some alternative candidate answers to her original question. This turn, which starts in line 3, is designed as a question, and thus requires E to offer another answer, which he does, in line 6. S then acknowledges E's answer in line 7 as being acceptable, by repeating the word 'gun' and mirroring his prosody.

A similar instance can be seen in the next example, fragment W2, where the child in the conversation is deaf. W, a 7-year-old deaf boy from an English-speaking family, is talking to his father. As was the case in fragment E2, a misunderstanding occurs when in line 2 W gives what F considers to be the wrong answer to his question in line 1. In this fragment, F uses the third turn in line 3 as the locus for 'repair' – he refutes W's answer to the question in line 2 by giving the 'right' answer, 'it was big'. The misunderstanding persists, as can be seen by W's elaboration of his original answer in line 4, 'it wasn't pink'. In line 5, F then indicates that he has understood the source of the misunderstanding – for W, who is lip-reading, 'big' and 'pink' have the same lip patterns. F then

```
   1   F:    was it big((asking about their hotel room))
   2   W:    no
->3   F:    it was big
   4   W:    it wasn't pink (.5)
   5   F:    no not pink  BI:::G   ((gestures))
   6   W:    big
   7   F:    ((nods))
   8   W:    yes
   9   F:    it was big
```

Figure 3.4 Fragment W2

adds a gesture to his rephrasing of the question in line 5. In line 8, W gives the 'right' answer, which is acknowledged by F in line 9. This type of lengthy repair sequence is frequently reported in conversations with deaf children and, indeed, in other conversations where one participant can be considered less competent – younger children, or people who have a communication disorder (Radford and Tarplee, 2000; Corrin, Tarplee and Wells, 2001; Ridley, Radford and Mahon, 2002).

The examples of data described thus far show a fairly natural and typical pattern of everyday talk between children and mature speakers. In both cases, some of the features of a child-directed speech style can be found: the mature speakers design their turns as 'test' questions; both speakers use the same language.

What about deaf children in EAL families? As can be seen in the next examples (Figures 3.5 and 3.6) the EAL parents talked to their deaf children in a very similar style to that described above, no matter what the home language of the family was, with one proviso: that the adult and the child speak the same language. The data fragments are from a conversation between Kh, a deaf boy aged 6 years 10 months and his father. Kh's parents stated that his first language is English, although their home language is Sylheti. His mother usually talks to him in Sylheti, and his father almost always talks to him in English. The example in Figure 3.5 is taken from a conversation between Kh and his father, F. The conversation is in English.

This sequence of talk is very similar to that presented in the above examples. In lines 5 and 7, each representing a third turn, F demonstrates that Kh's answers are perfectly acceptable and correct. It is of interest to note here that in line 3, F responds to Kh's clarification request in line 2 by saying 'mm' with a falling intonation. That this response indeed clarifies the question asked in line 1 is evidenced in line 4, where Kh gives his answer. F then acknowledges the answer in line 5. F's use of the 'mm' here is warranted by Kh's request for clarification and it promotes further interaction (Schegloff, 1984).

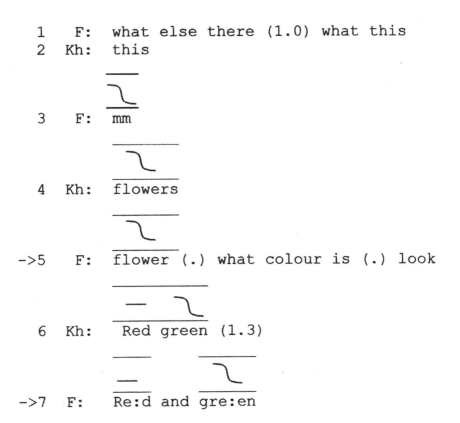

```
1   F:   what else there (1.0) what this
2   Kh:  this
                    ⌐‾‾⌐
                      ⟍_

3   F:   mm
                  ⌐‾‾‾‾⌐
                    ⟍_

4   Kh:  flowers
                ⌐‾‾‾‾‾⌐
                   ⟍_

->5  F:   flower (.) what colour is (.) look
                 ⌐‾‾‾‾‾‾‾‾‾⌐
                  —      ⟍_

6   Kh:  Red green (1.3)
            ⌐‾‾⌐         ⌐‾‾⌐
             —            ⟍_

->7  F:   Re:d and gre:en
```

Figure 3.5 Fragment Khf1


```
1 M:     say what the man's doing ((both Kh and M look
         down at a page in Kh's school reading book))
                              ⌐‾‾‾⌐
                               ⟍_

2 Kh:    oh playing with the (.) boxing
           ⌐‾⌐
            —

3 M:     mm
               ⌐‾‾‾⌐
                ⟍_

4 Kh:    boxing
         (2.9)
```

Figure 3.6 Fragment Khm1

In all of the data fragments presented so far, two features are consistently apparent:

- both speakers are using the same language
- the typical three-turn labelling sequence with expected design of the third turn is evident.

CA analysis of the conversations shows that they are locally managed and interactionally managed. However, there was one set of conversations in which a striking difference was noticeable. These were the conversations between Sylheti-speaking mothers and their English-speaking deaf sons.

When examples of this data were analysed, it became apparent that although the talk was obviously locally managed, that is, each speaker took a turn in the correct place, there was a consistent departure from the typical pattern described above. Obviously the participants were not speaking the same language: the mothers spoke Sylheti, the deaf boys spoke English. But careful analysis then revealed a second subtle and important difference. This was that in the 'talking about pictures activity', the participants revealed that their talk was not interactionally managed, that is, the data did not show that intersubjectivity had been achieved. What was striking about this finding was the frequency with which it occurred in the conversations between the mothers and their sons.

The difference was typified in the way the third turn in the sequence was designed by the mothers. As will be seen in the examples given below, no lexical or phonetic checks were displayed – there was no repetition or partial repetition of the prior turn and the intonation patterns of answer and receipt were quite different. The third turn locus was not used to signal either overt or implicit display of understanding.

The first example is from a conversation between Kh and his mother, M (Figure 3.6). This is the same deaf boy as was seen talking to his father in fragment KhF 1 above. Kh speaks English and M speaks Sylheti in the interaction. Once again, the transcription shows that words translated into colloquial English from Sylheti are printed in italics.

M takes her turn in line 3 (the third turn of the sequence) but she does not use a word here, hence there is no lexical clue to her response to Kh's answer (line 2) to the question (line 1). Neither does M give a prosodic cue to her response in line 3, as there is no matching of her prosody to his prior turn. Evidence that there is some difficulty with M's turn in line 3 is found in line 4, where Kh repeats his answer 'boxing'. However, M does not take another turn, and the talk ends with a long pause. No check on understanding is displayed by M. Arguably, it is possible that a misunderstanding has arisen and the opportunity to resolve that misunderstanding has not been taken.

A similar conclusion can be drawn from the next example (Figure 3.7) which is taken from a conversation between A, a 7-year-old deaf boy

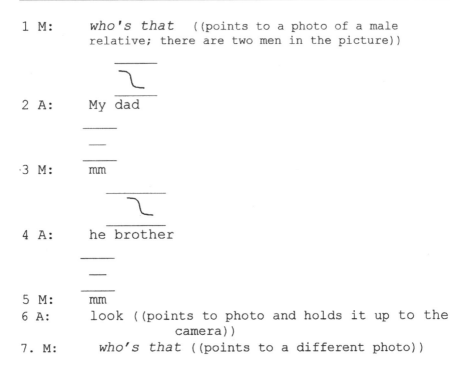

```
1 M:      who's that   ((points to a photo of a male
                        relative; there are two men in the picture))


2 A:      My dad


·3 M:      mm


4 A:      he brother


5 M:      mm
6 A:      look ((points to photo and holds it up to the
                       camera))
7. M:     who's that ((points to a different photo))
```

Figure 3.7 Fragment Am1

and his mother, M. As was the case for Kh's family, A's mother said that his first language is English. She always speaks Sylheti to A. In fragment AM1, A and his mother M are talking about some family photos.

In response to the question in line 1, A has offered a candidate answer in line 2, 'my dad', but appears to offer another answer in line 4 'he brother'. M takes her turns in lines 3 and 5, but what she says are not words, so there is no overt lexical component to her turns which could provide a clue about her understanding of A's answers to her question in line 1. There is also no evidence of the kind of prosodic matching which has previously been taken as indicative of affirmation of the adequacy or 'rightness' of the answer in either lines 3 or 5. Although M has responded to his answers in lines 3 and 5, it would seem by looking to the camera being operated by the researcher, he appears to be seeking another response. The sequence of talk is ended when M turns to another photo and asks a 'starter' question in line 8.

As was the case for fragment KhM1, it would seem that neither the prosody nor the utterance itself appears to explicitly indicate under-standing, in contrast to the examples of talk involving W and Kh (see fragments W1, KhF1 and KhF2) where there was always some lexical or prosodic reference (or both) to the prior turn. Before discussing the implications of this analysis, one final example will be given.

Fragment AM2 (Figure 3.8) illustrates this further. In this fragment, M points to the picture of the uncle and says 'mama' with a rising intonation

```
1 M:      mama*? ((M points to a man in the
          photo. Other family members including A's
          mother are also pictured.))
2 A:      (A looks down at the photo))
```

```
          mama (.) my (.) mama ((pointing to the same
                                        photo))
```

```
 3 M:     mm
 4 A:     that my (.) THAT my mum ((looks up at camera;
          holds the same photo up to the camera; points
          to his mother's picture))
```

```
5 M:     mm
    (2.3)
```

*This word, mama, is the kinship term in Sylheti meaning maternal uncle (STAR, 2001).

Figure 3.8 Fragment Am2

as though she were asking a question. In line 2, A answers using the same word, 'mama'. M's third turn (line 3), does not indicate how she may be understanding A's answer – she says 'mm' with flat intonation. That this could be problematic for A is displayed in line 4 when he involves the camera in the interaction and uses the English word 'mum' to refer to the photo. In line 5, M then gives another 'mm' as her next turn, once again not overtly displaying whether or not she understands. M's receipts of A's turns are all similar, no matter what A's prior utterance was. She says 'mm'. That there has been an unresolved misunderstanding of the word 'mama'[1] seems evident to the analyst. Throughout the conversation before and after this segment, A's mother uses the word 'amma' (meaning 'mummy') to refer to herself, and never uses 'mama' to mean 'mummy'. From the way in which she designs her turns, it would appear that A's mother has not registered that A might have misunderstood the kinship term 'mama' meaning maternal uncle. By saying 'mama my mama' in line 2, A indicates that he is referring to the picture of his mother, and not his uncle. He displays his meaning again, by referring the picture to the camera, and using the English term, 'mum' in line 4.

The analysis of this fragment tells a similar story to that told about fragments KhM1 and AM1: the mothers are seen to display local management of the question–answer labelling sequences in their conversation by completing the three-turn structural pattern. However, they do not use the third turn locus to indicate understanding. Arguably, therefore, the systematic opportunity to attend to any possible misunderstanding arising from the first or second turns is not taken up in the third turn. Their use of 'mm' (which is neither Sylheti nor English) is unlike the 'mm' used by Kh's father in fragment KhF1, and it is also unlike the 'mm hm' in story progression (Sacks, 1995 [1968] and the 'uhus' and other 'continuers' which are described by Schegloff (1982) as tokens presented to the speaker by the listener to acknowledge that an extended turn is under way. Without displaying overt or implicit understanding, the 'mms' here put pressure on the deaf child to do more.

Conclusions

What sense can be made of this data? Although only a few fragments from the extensive corpus have been discussed here, it is possible to offer some preliminary conclusions. The first concerns the language used by family members to their deaf children. The examples given clearly show that when the mothers and their deaf children are not speaking the same language, the talk is different from that observed in the data when the same language is spoken. In the latter case, conversation unfolds in a normal way, as was seen in the talk between Kh and his father, and W and his father. But in the talk between A and Kh and their mothers there is little evidence of the overt checks on understanding and opportunities for resolving misunderstandings so commonly found in the talk between deaf children and hearing adults who speak the same language. Such checks could provide the deaf children with the input from which they could enhance their language skills. Both the mothers and the deaf children have a very difficult communicative task: the mothers are trying to understand the boys' idiosyncratic English which is sometimes made more difficult because of deafness-related speech intelligibility problems. The kind of labelling responses that we believe foster language development in this circumstance do not materialize in the way they did when, for example, Kh and his father talk to each other in English. Similarly, when misunderstandings occur, fixing them up could mean the mothers engaging in lengthy repair sequences (like that seen in fragment W1) which in themselves represent risking further misunderstanding and communication 'failure'. The deaf children's communication task is also difficult: their language skills are mainly in English, and they do not have the Sylheti words that could facilitate their communication with their mothers.

Looked at from a western child-centred perspective, the type of talk shown in fragments KhM1; AM1 and AM2 could imply a language environment for A and Kh that may not provide the language learning opportunities thought to be necessary for a deaf child. However, it is unrealistic to expect the mothers to have a command of English that would enable them to provide and to take advantage of such opportunities. If Sylheti was being spoken by both mother and child, there would probably be a much better chance of normal interaction unfolding. Clearly, asking these mothers to speak any language other than their home language to their deaf children can lead to real problems in communication within the family (Ahmad et al, 1998).

An obvious implication of this conclusion has to do with intervention by professionals in the deaf child's life, and with the crucial question of which language should be used at home. The evidence from this study supports the notion that the family should be encouraged, with the employment of appropriate resources where necessary, to use their home language with their deaf child. Unless there are realistic opportunities for family members to learn English quickly and appropriately without undue expense, asking them to speak English could be a course of action which may fail all the key players: the families, the deaf child and the well-intentioned professionals. The frustration that can be engendered in all parties concerned is encapsulated in the following comment made by a deaf man of Indian origin who took part in Sharma and Love's study (1991):

> I can speak a little English but I'd like to *speak* Gugerati. I asked for speech therapy in Gugerati but only English is available. I want to speak Gugerati so I can talk to my mum and so that I can make devotions in the temple. I asked the social worker but she said my mum must learn to sign. But my mum's too old to learn English. If only I'd been brought up to speak Gugerati we could communicate.' (Sharma and Love, 1991:9)

A further implication for intervention has been illuminated by the data. This concerns the way in which of professionals working with deaf children regard 'fostering language development'. The approach centres around early intervention, in which the parents are considered to be partners with the professionals in a programme of actively encouraging language development for the child, loosely based on the child-directed speech style approach (Pressman et al, 1999). How can intervention in the early years of a deaf child's life be made appropriate for EAL families like those discussed in this chapter? We have to question the beginning of the therapeutic endeavour which starts with an establishment of trust between the professionals and the parents, based on a mutual belief that a deaf child can indeed become a communicator (Turner, 1996). In this, both parties could be operating from positions of relative ignorance about each other's standpoint: the professional may not have much understanding of the deaf child's family culture, and the family, for its part, could equally not have insight into the therapist's culture of intervention. Unrealistic expectations on both sides could stall the process. Further complications can ensue when the intervention has to be conducted via a translator – the delicate (and easily broken) web of understanding that is needed for translated intervention to work properly has been well documented elsewhere (CICHS, 1995; Leather and Wirz, 1996; RCSLT, 1998; Silvera and Kapasi, 2000). The insight provided by the data here points to the need to question the appropriateness of our strategies, and not to take anything for granted. When issues to do with language, culture and deafness are combined in one family, the integrity of the professionals is tested to the limit.

The final comments to be made here concern the compelling reasons why CA is a suitable choice of methodology for investigating interactions with deaf people and with deaf children in particular. This data-driven approach emphasizes the detailed description of observable behaviour, enabling a move away from the 'deficiency' model (Webster, 1986) within which deafness continues to be regarded. From a practical point of view, it can be said that CA descriptions of conversations with deaf children may promote understanding of the underlying components of the communication difficulties that exist when deaf children and hearing adults converse without prejudice. It is hoped that such understanding will inform rehabilitation strategies and reveal further areas for research.

Appendix

Transcription notation

The notational system in these transcriptions is based on that detailed by Levinson (1983:369–370) and by Atkinson and Heritage (1984: ix–xvi).

Simultaneous utterances	[[ ]]
Overlapping utterances	[
Contiguous utterances	=
Intervals between utterances	(10ths of a second)
	(.) less than 0.5 s
Lengthening	:::::
Loudness	CAPS
Quiet	° °
Aspirations/inhalations	(hh)
Vocalizations	((cough))
Details of conversational scene	((phone rings))
Transcriptionist doubt	( ) or (unintelligible)
Flat intonation	‾
Falling intonation	⌐_

Audiological information

- W has a severe-profound bilateral sensori-neural hearing loss diagnosed at 11 months following meningitis.
- Kh has a prelingual moderate–severe bilateral mixed hearing loss.
- A has a prelingual profound bilateral sensori-neural hearing loss.

Chapter 4
Spoken communication between deaf and hearing pupils

JULIAN LLOYD

A recent estimate suggested that approximately 85% of deaf children in British schools are now taught in mainstream (Lynas, Lewis and Hopwood, 1997; Watson and Parsons, 1998). The trend towards mainstream integration, and the growing practice of providing in-class support rather than withdrawal, means that increasingly more deaf pupils are being taught alongside their hearing peers (Watson and Parsons, 1998). One of the main arguments that is used to support policies of inclusion is that integration is conducive to academic achievement and social and communicative development in children with special needs (McNamara, 1997). For deaf children, however, this proposition has not been proven in the research literature (Lloyd, 1999a). Relatively little research has focused on interaction between school-age deaf and hearing children (Gregory and Knight, 1998; Lloyd, 1999a; Lloyd, Lieven and Arnold, 2001).

This chapter reports a study that focuses on spoken communication between deaf and hearing pupils. The aim of the chapter is to consider ways in which hearing peers might contribute to the communicative and academic development of deaf pupils. First, the chapter draws on developmental psychology, to develop a theoretical framework for the study. Then, a study of spoken communication between deaf and hearing children during a structured communication task is reported. The aim of the study was to identify communicative strategies that might support communication between deaf and hearing pupils, focusing specifically on their clarification strategies (see Lloyd, 1999b). It was hoped that the study would give some indication of the types of roles that hearing peers may play in the communicative and academic development of deaf children. The chapter ends with recommendations for future research that might make the nature of these roles clearer.

Interaction and child development

Studies by Wood and his colleagues on tutoring have provided a starting point for the present research (Wood, Bruner and Ross, 1976; Wood, Wood and Middleton, 1978; Wood et al, 1995; Wood and O'Malley, 1996). By studying the role of adult instruction in child learning, these authors developed a 'scaffolding' metaphor to describe the types of adult behaviour that can support and facilitate children's problem-solving skills (Wood, Bruner and Ross, 1976; also see Wood, 1988, 1991, 1998). They observed mothers instructing their 4- to 5-year-old children to build a pyramid from wooden blocks. Five levels of instruction were identified, and these became progressively more controlling, ranging from general verbal encouragement through to direct demonstration of specific actions. Generally, the more controlling an instruction, the greater the extent to which it directs the child's behaviour in the task. These investigators found that effective instruction involved giving instructions that were *contingent* on the child's successes and failures; 'that is, by making any help given conditional upon the child's understandings of previous levels of instruction' (Wood, 1988:79). This finding led Wood (1991) to define the 'the *process* of effective instruction as the contingent control of learning' (p. 105).

Theoretically, the work of Wood and his colleagues has its roots in Vygotsky's (1978) Zone of Proximal Development (ZPD), which emphasizes the importance of social interaction to child development. According to Vygotsky, there are two levels of development: an actual level – that which a child can achieve independently; and a potential level – that which a child can achieve through collaboration with a more experienced partner. The ZPD is the distance between the actual and potential developmental levels, or the difference between unassisted and assisted performance (Tharp and Gallimore, 1991). Vygotsky argued that the level of achievement displayed by a child under the guidance of a more experienced partner may eventually be achieved independently. For Vygotsky instruction by a more skilled partner is the factor that facilitates development (Wood, 1991; 1998; Durkin, 1995; Light and Littleton, 1999).

The term 'scaffolding' was first used to describe the types of adult behaviour that supported children's problem-solving skills in an experimental task, but it has since been used more generally in the literature to describe the types of interaction and communication which support children's learning and development. Attention has also turned to interactions between children, to determine whether scaffolding processes occur (Light and Littleton, 1999). Wood (1998) suggests that peer interaction often involves an element of informal teaching, which he views as an essential feature of human behaviour that often occurs without 'teachers' being aware that they are 'teaching'. Rogoff (1990, 1991) has taken a similar stance, using the term 'guided participation' to describe the process by which children learn through 'shared cultural activities' (Rogoff, 1990:98).

The literature suggests that children are less successful than adults at scaffolding other children's learning. Ellis and Rogoff (1986) compared 8- to 9-year-olds with adults as tutors of 6- to 7-year-olds during classification tasks. They found that, in addition to problems with the classification of task items, the child tutors experienced problems with communicating task instructions, assessing learner needs, and organizing their instruction. This finding led them to conclude that 'instructional interaction is a problem-solving situation for both teacher and learner' (Ellis and Rogoff, 1986:303). They did suggest, however, that the observed behaviour may have been more typical of that particular experimental task than tutoring in naturalistic contexts, acknowledging that children may be more effective tutors in naturalistic contexts.

Other commentators have suggested that children's ability to scaffold other children's learning improves with age (Cooper, Marquis and Edward, 1986; Wood et al, 1995; Wood and O'Malley, 1996). In a study of same-age tutoring using the pyramid task, Wood et al (1995) found that most of their 7-year-olds, some of their 5-year-olds, but none of their 3-year-olds could teach contingently. Their results showed significant changes in tutoring strategies, verbal instruction, and contingency of teaching at the three ages.

Regarding learning in the classroom, Cooper, Marquis and Edward (1986) have argued that scaffolding is more likely to occur when children aged 10 years and above are tutors. They suggest that the inability to provide adequate scaffolding in younger children may be attributable to limitations in both cognitive and discourse skills. However, these authors do identify ways in which younger children provide assistance for each other in learning situations, which they term 'pacing episodes' (p. 275). For example, young children provide 'attentional anchoring' for each other in the classroom, when working side-by-side but on different problems in their work books.

Peer interaction has attracted considerable attention from Neo-Piagetian scholars (e.g. Doise and Mugny, 1984). Piaget (1932) argued that peer interaction plays an important role in overcoming some of the limitations of pre-operational thinking, particularly egocentrism. Due to differences in power relations and status between adult-child and peer interactions, children are more likely to try to resolve differences of points of view when they occur in interactions with peers. Piaget argued that exposure to, and the resolution of, differing viewpoints is an important factor in a child's cognitive development. A strand of research by Doise and his colleagues suggested that collaboration between children who had different perspectives on the same problem appeared to facilitate cognitive gains in these children. These authors argued that 'socio-cognitive conflict', the experience of encountering these different perspectives, was the factor that facilitated the cognitive gains (see Doise and Mugny, 1984).

Light and his colleagues have made a major contribution to the study of peer interaction and its role in cognitive development by identifying some of the interactive and communicative processes that support cognitive development. A major aspect of this body of work was the use of computer-based tasks as a context for peer collaboration. These researchers have consistently demonstrated that collaboration with peers facilitates problem-solving skills in comparison to individual performance (see Light and Littleton, 1999 for a review). These authors' findings have suggested that processes such as dialogue, negotiation, planning, joint decision making, and the co-construction of knowledge and ideas play important roles in collaborative learning. This programme of research has extended Neo-Piagetian accounts of the role of socio-cognitive conflict in cognitive development by highlighting the point that interactive and communicative processes can play important roles: 'it is not simply exposure to solutions that differ from your own, but actually being forced to engage with them in some way, which fosters improved performance' (Light and Littleton, 1999:19). The present study examines spoken communication between deaf and hearing pupils during a structured task to try to begin to determine some of the communicative processes that might support collaborative learning between deaf and hearing pupils.

Interaction between deaf and hearing children

Interaction between deaf and hearing children of school age has received relatively little attention in the research literature. The main findings of the research on children of pre-school and primary school age were reviewed by Lloyd (1999a) and Lloyd, Lieven and Arnold (2001) and can be summarized as follows:

• both deaf and hearing children prefer to interact with peers of the same hearing status
• both deaf and hearing children appear to be more successful at interacting with children with whom they are familiar
• deaf children with better linguistic skills are more likely to interact with their hearing peers than are those with less linguistic ability

Other research has focused on the quantity of speech that hearing peers elicit from deaf children in comparison to other communication partners. Niver and Schery (1994) compared hearing peers with mothers as communication partners of deaf children, finding that deaf children spoke more to their mothers than to peers. More recently, Lloyd, Lieven and Arnold (2001) compared hearing peers with teachers as communication partners of deaf children. These authors found that deaf children had a tendency to communicate more with teachers than peers, but they tended to use longer speaking turns when talking to peers. A qualitative analysis suggested that this pattern of results may have been influenced by differences in the frequency of question–answer sequences between the teacher–child and child–child sessions. The deaf children studied by Lloyd, Lieven and Arnold (2001) tended to provide minimal answers in response to teacher questions, which supports the findings of Wood and his colleagues in their studies of teacher–child interaction (see Wood et al, 1986). In the child–child sessions, however, question–answer sequences were rare, with the deaf children tending to use a higher proportion of declarative utterances (i.e. comments and statements) than in the teacher–child sessions (also see Lloyd, 1999a). So, the deaf children were proportionally more likely to use longer speaking turns with peers than teachers.

Research on interaction between deaf and hearing pupils of secondary-school age has attempted to determine whether hearing peers can contribute to the development of deaf children in the classroom. Burley, Gutkin, and Nauman (1994) showed that a hearing peer could successfully tutor a deaf pupil to acquire certain mathematics skills, concluding that peer tutoring may be used profitably in the mainstreaming of deaf children. Miller (1995) examined cooperative learning between deaf and hearing pupils and found that, in comparison to traditional teaching methods, cooperative learning had a positive effect on the way in which the deaf children engaged in conversational interaction.

So, previous studies of interaction between deaf and hearing pupils have suggested that hearing peers can play facilitative roles in both the academic and communicative development of deaf pupils. Nevertheless, it is reasonable to suggest that collaboration between deaf and hearing pupils may sometimes be problematic. One factor that might lead to problems in collaborative situations is that deaf and hearing children rely primarily on different perceptual systems. Deaf children tend to rely more heavily on their visual systems than hearing children, who in turn tend to take a 'simultaneous visual-auditory approach' (Jamieson, 1994:168). Deaf and hearing children may therefore be taking different perceptual approaches to a shared problem during collaborative tasks. To the author's knowledge, no research has specifically addressed this issue, but a study of mother–child interaction by Jamieson (1994) gives some indication of the kinds of problems that might arise in collaborative situations between deaf and hearing children.

Jamieson (1994) compared the instructional discourse of deaf and hearing mothers of deaf children using the Wood, Bruner and Ross (1976) pyramid task. She found that deaf mothers used adaptive strategies that took into consideration the deaf child's need to give and receive information 'in a sequential visual manner' (p. 167). They used more comments and directives than hearing mothers, for example, which require 'far less breaking off and re-establishing visual contact with the child than . . . questioning' (p. 167). When deaf children made errors or misunderstood, hearing mothers tended to rely on repetition as a discourse strategy, rather than using 'an altered, visual approach' (p. 168). Jamieson suggests that the behaviour of hearing mothers derives from their 'simultaneous visual-auditory approach' (p. 168), and that the behaviour is less conducive to the cognitive and linguistic development of deaf children than the altered, visual approach of the deaf mothers.

Considering that children are generally less skilful than adults at instructing other children (see above), and their less developed cognitive and discourse skills make it less likely that they will be able to use adaptive strategies to overcome the difficulties of approaching a shared problem while relying primarily on different perceptual systems, it is easy to envisage that problems may arise during collaborative activities between deaf and hearing children.

The communication of route directions between deaf children and their hearing peers

As discussed, relatively little research has focused on interaction between school-age deaf and hearing pupils. The present study examines spoken communication between deaf and hearing pupils during a structured task to try to determine communication strategies that might support collaborative learning between deaf and hearing pupils. The study aimed to determine whether deaf–hearing dyads use adaptive communication strategies in such a task, or whether they use similar communication strategies to hearing dyads.

As the study aimed to systematically examine negotiation and the exchange of information between deaf and hearing pupils, it was considered that a structured task with an intrinsic goal was required. Studies by Peter Lloyd (1991, 1992, 1993) and Anderson and her colleagues (e.g. Anderson et al, 1991) have suggested that map tasks provide a good context for studying negotiation between children. One of the main advantages of map tasks is that they are goal-directed, and participants and researchers both know the goal. From the participants' viewpoint, having a goal means there is intrinsic value to successful communication. From the researchers' viewpoint, knowing the participants' goal eliminates some of the subjectivity when interpreting their utterances. The researchers' knowledge of referents also permits objective decisions about effective communication, ambiguity, etc. and permits the measurement of successful communication (Anderson et al, 1991). For the present study a map task based on that of Peter Lloyd (1991) was developed.

Table 4.1 Categories of clarification requests used in the map task

Category	Examples
Non-specific requests for repetition	(1) L: 'what?' (2) L: 'pardon?' (3) L: 'huh?' (4) L: 'eh?' (5) L: 'say that again'

Specific requests for repetition	(1) S: 'then number three castle'
	    L: 'which castle?'
	    S: 'the third castle'
	(2) S: 'up to the garage with the four garage on it'
	    L: 'with the what?'
	    S: 'four garage'

Specific requests for confirmation	(1) S: 'turn right with two trees'
	    L: 'right?'
	    S: 'yeah'
	(2) S: 'go to the fire station with four doors'
	    L: 'got four?'
	    S: 'four doors'

Specific requests for specification	S: 'then straight on through the castle' L: 'which castle?' S: 'the one straight ahead of you'

Potential requests for elaboration	(1) S: 'one fireman'
	    L: 'how many doors in the fire station?'
	    S: 'four'
	(2) S: 'the bus goes to the church'
	    L: 'what colour?'
	    S: 'blue'

Potential request for confirmation	(1) S: 'turn left to the first hospital'
	    L: 'with two ambulances?'
	    S: 'yeah'
	(2) S: 'then it carries up then it turns left'
	    L: 'what's got one big tree?'
	    S: 'yeah'

Potential request for specification (prs)	(1) S: 'blue little flag yellow little flag are same'
	    L: 'is it the third castle or the fourth?'
	    S: 'erm number two'
	(2) S: 'left'
	    L: 'got four garage got two garage?'
	    S: 'four garage'

As the study aimed to identify communication strategies that can lead to successful communication between deaf and hearing children, a logical focal point was clarification strategies, which are an important aspect of successful communication (Lloyd, 1999b). The present study focuses on the use of clarification requests. These are devices that listeners use when they have misheard or misunderstood a speaker's message. Three main types of clarification request have been identified: *non-specific*, *specific*, and *potential* (Lloyd, 1992). Examples of each type are given in Table 4.1.

- **Non-specific requests for repetition.** Non-specific requests for repetition are general requests that give no indication as to why the speaker's utterance was deficient.
- **Specific requests.** Specific requests relate to the form or content of the speaker's original utterance, and so they are more informative than non-specific requests because they indicate the source of the breakdown in communication (Lloyd, 1992).
- **Potential requests.** Potential requests introduce 'information not contained in the previous utterance' (Lloyd, 1992:369); that is, information that was missing from the speaker's previous utterance but which was 'potentially available' (Lloyd, 1992: 362). In (2) under *potential requests for elaboration* in Table 4.1, for example, the speaker makes no reference to the colour of the church, but the listener introduces colour to try to identify the correct referent. Potential requests therefore demand more work by the listener than non-specific and specific requests.

Earlier studies of deaf children's use of clarification requests have suggested that, in comparison to typically developing children, deaf children are more likely to use non-specific rather than specific requests (see Lloyd, 1999b for a review). This is generally interpreted to mean that some deaf children are delayed in their acquisition of clarification strategies. Alternatively, Jeanes, Nienhuys and Rickards (2000) have suggested that an increased use of clarification requests overall, and especially the increased use of non-specific requests for repetition and specific requests for confirmation (see Table 4.1) by deaf children who are communicating orally, are adaptive strategies due to their 'imperfect oral communication reception'. Following Jeanes, Nienhuys and Rickards (2000), the present study aimed to examine whether deaf–hearing dyads would use adaptive clarification strategies, resulting from either the deaf children's difficulty in perceiving spoken communication, or difficulties that the hearing peers might have with communicating with a deaf child.

Method

Participants

A total of 104 children participated (26 deaf and 78 hearing children). The 26 deaf children had ages ranging from 7;4 to 11;9 years (M = 9;7; SD = 1;4). Their mean better ear average hearing loss (BEA HL) was 92.57 dB (SD = 14.46; range = 71–121). All had prelinguistic hearing losses (defined as congenital hearing losses or those acquired before 2 years of age). Of the 26 deaf children, 24 were from oral schools and 2 from schools that used Total Communication. Each deaf child selected a hearing friend from one of his or her mainstream classes to act as a partner in the map task. The peers had a mean age of 9;5 years (SD = 1.2; range = 7;6–11;5). A control group of hearing dyads was matched for age and sex with the deaf–hearing dyads. The controls had a mean age of 9;6 years (SD = 1;2; range = 7;4–11;2).

The task

See Figure 4.1 and Table 4.2 for details of the map task.

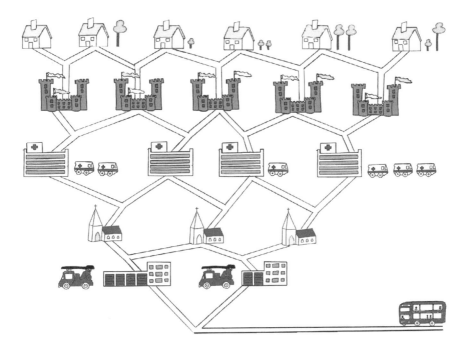

Figure 4.1 The map

Table 4.2 Buildings that were used as landmarks in the map task

Row	Type of building	No. in row	Critical attribute
A	Fire station	2	Number of garage doors (4 or 2)
B	Church	3	Colour of door (green, yellow or blue)
C	Hospital	4	Number of ambulances (2, 0, 1 or 3)
D	Castle	5	Placement of a yellow and a blue flag
E	House	6	Number and size of trees

Procedure

The children sat opposite each other at a table, with a small cardboard barrier between them. This prevented them from seeing each other's map, while allowing lip-reading and the use of gestures. The task was introduced using a standardized script and warm-up exercises. The speaker's map had a route marked on it and the listener's task was to reproduce the route through negotiation with the speaker. The participants alternated as speakers and listeners over 6 trials (routes), so that each child had 3 attempts as 'speaker' (giving directions) and 3 as 'listener' (following directions). In the first trial 11 of the deaf children acted as speakers and 15 as listeners. This was to have been counter-balanced, but two schools dropped out of the study at a late stage of data collection. Videotapes of the sessions were transcribed and analysed.

Analysis

Speaker and listener performance

The analytical procedure was adapted from P. Lloyd (1991, 1992, 1993). Two measures were used to assess speaker and listener performance: 'message adequacy' (speaker) and 'correct identification of landmarks' (listener). The unit of analysis was 'move', the dialogue involved in getting from one landmark to the next on the map. Each dyad negotiated 30 moves (5 moves in 6 trials).

Message adequacy was determined from the standpoint of the speaker. Each move on the map involved a choice between two alternatives if standard map conventions were being followed. An adequate message was defined as one that discriminated between the two alternatives for that move. Adequacy was further defined to include information that emerged from the dialogue between the participants that was sufficient to allow the target to be identified. It could therefore relate to more than one utterance, or to the contribution of both participants. Listener performance was measured in terms of the number of landmarks correctly identified regardless of message adequacy, and so this measure includes fortuitous successes.

It should be noted that 'adequate message' and 'landmarks correctly identified' reflect the performance of the dyad more than its individual members, as speaker performance has an influence on listener performance, and vice versa. For example, a speaker who is not yet certain about the difference between left and right, but tries to use a directional strategy without providing any additional information (e.g. by saying 'go to the church on the left' when the church is actually on the right), may inevitably cause the listener to select the wrong landmark. Similarly, a speaker might provide necessary information following a request for further information by the listener. This type of task does not give a true indication of individual ability because the dyad members can influence each other's performance, and therefore this analysis focuses primarily on the performance of dyads.

Clarification requests

Clarification requests by listeners were categorized according to the coding scheme shown in Table 4.1.

Gestures

A fine-grained analysis of non-verbal communication was not made, but gestures that were used to supplement spoken instructions (i.e. those that encoded the critical elements of the message) were examined (e.g. holding up two fingers when saying 'two ambulances', using gestures to help to discriminate between 'big' and 'small', or pointing 'left' or 'right'). Gestures such as nodding or shaking of the head were not included in this analysis because it was often unclear as to whether these were directed to the other child.

Results and discussion

Message adequacy and landmarks correctly identified: a comparison of the deaf-hearing and control dyads

First, the communicative performance of the deaf-hearing and control dyads was compared. The mean percentage of adequate messages given when speakers, and percentage of landmarks correctly identified when listeners, are shown in Table 4.3. The percentage scores were transformed with the arcsine transform to eliminate floor and ceiling effects in the following statistical comparisons (Howell, 1992). When comparing group means, it was found that the control dyads performed more successfully than the deaf–hearing dyads, giving significantly more adequate messages ($t(50) = 2.64$, $p < 0.02$) and correctly identifying significantly more landmarks ($t(50) = 5.01$, $p < 0.01$) than the deaf–hearing dyads. No order effects were found; whether the deaf child was speaker first or listener first made no difference to scores of message adequacy or landmarks correctly identified.

When the deaf–hearing dyads were compared as speakers and listeners, it was found that the deaf–hearing dyads performed better as speakers than listeners ($t(25) = 3.03$, $p<0.01$), suggesting that some members of the deaf–hearing dyads may have found it difficult to hear or interpret their partner's instructions.

Table 4.3 Mean percentages (SD; range) of adequate messages (speakers) and landmarks correctly identified (listeners)

	Deaf–hearing	Controls
Adequate messages[a]	89.36 (11.43; 56.67–100)	96.15 (4.96; 83.33–100)
Landmarks identified[b]	82.31 (16.62; 46.67–100	97.05 (5.76; 80–100)

[a]Controls higher than deaf–hearing, $p < 0.02$.
[b]Controls higher than deaf–hearing, $p < 0.01$.

The study was also designed to examine whether communication between deaf and hearing children changed over time. Micro-analytic techniques were used to examine the children's communication in successive attempts to negotiate routes. For clarity the members of the dyads were subcategorized:

- **First speakers** (FS) were the participants who acted as speakers in the first trial. They were speakers in trials 1, 3, and 5 and listeners in trials 2, 4, and 6.
- **First listeners** (FL) were listeners in trials 1, 3, and 5 and speakers in trials 2, 4, and 6.

Figure 4.2 shows the percentage of adequate messages given in the three trials in which FS were speaker. Regarding message adequacy, FS in both the deaf–hearing and control dyads improved over three trials. As speakers, FS in the deaf–hearing dyads were performing at a lower level than the controls in the 1st trial, but were performing at a similar level to the controls in the third trial.

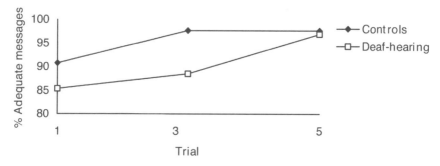

Figure 4.2 Percentage of adequate messages for FS over three trials

Figure 4.3 shows the percentage of adequate messages given in the three trials in which FL were speaker. In the first trial FL in the deaf–hearing dyads were performing at a lower level than FL in the control dyads. The performance of FL in the controls dipped in the third trial, but FL in the deaf–hearing dyads continued to improve over the three trials, so that both groups were performing at a more similar level as speakers in the third than in the first trial.

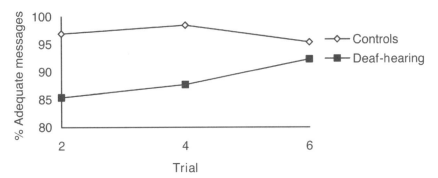

Figure 4.3 Percentage of adequate messages for FL over three trials.

Figure 4.4 shows the percentage of landmarks correctly identified in the three trials in which FL were listener. As listeners, there was a large difference between FL in the deaf–hearing and control dyads in the first trial, but both were performing at a more similar level in the third trial.

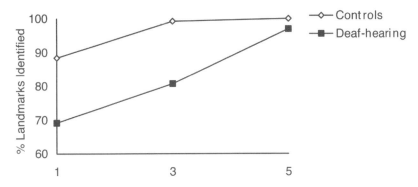

Figure 4.4 Percentage of landmarks correctly identified by FL over three trials

Figure 4.5 shows the percentage of landmarks correctly identified in the three trials in which FS were listeners. FS in the deaf–hearing dyads improved over the three trials. In the first trial there was a large difference between FS in the deaf–hearing and control dyads in the percentage of landmarks correctly identified. FS in the control dyads were effectively at ceiling level throughout the three trials. As listeners, FS in the deaf–hearing and control dyads were performing at a more similar level in the third than in the first trial.

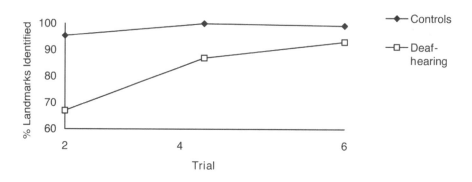

Figure 4.5 Percentage of landmarks correctly identified by FS over three trials

In summary, Figures 4.2–4.5 show that the deaf–hearing dyads improved as speakers and listeners over three trials. In the first trial as both speakers and listeners, the performance of the deaf–hearing dyads was inferior to that of the controls. By the third trial, however, the performance of the deaf–hearing and control dyads was more similar regarding the percentage of adequate messages and landmarks correctly identified. It can therefore be argued that the deaf–hearing dyads performed better as speakers and listeners than was suggested by their mean scores of message adequacy and correct selection of landmarks. These findings illustrate an advantage of using micro-analyses in the study of children's communication. The improvements in the deaf–hearing dyads' communication was not shown through the comparison of group means.

Clarification requests: deaf–hearing dyads compared with the controls

The frequency and mean number of clarification requests made by the deaf-hearing and control dyads is shown in Table 4.4. The deaf–hearing dyads made significantly more clarification requests than the controls

Table 4.4 Frequency and mean number (SD; range) of clarification requests made by the deaf–hearing and control dyads

	Deaf–hearing	Controls
Frequency	422	221
Mean number[a]	16.23 (14.42; 0–63)	8.5 (9.91; 0–43)

[a]Deaf–hearing higher than controls, $p < 0.05$.

$(t(50) = 2.25, p < 0.05)$. The higher use of clarification requests by the deaf–hearing dyads in comparison to the controls may be viewed as an adaptive strategy, resulting from the communication difficulties experienced by their deaf and hearing members.

Table 4.5 Percentage distribution of non-specific, specific and potential clarification requests for the deaf–hearing and control dyads

	Deaf–hearing	Controls
Non-specific	11.37	0.9
Specific	43.13	45.5
Potential	45.5	54.75

Table 4.5 shows the percentage distribution of non-specific, specific and potential clarification requests made by the deaf–hearing and control dyads. A higher proportion of the deaf–hearing dyads' clarification requests was non-specific requests compared to the controls.

Table 4.6 Mean number (SD; range) of non-specific, specific and potential clarification requests made by the deaf–hearing and control dyads

	Deaf–hearing	Controls
Non-specific requests for repetition[a]	1.85 (2.43; 0–9)	0.08 (0.39; 0–2)
Specific requests[b]	7.0 (6.18; 0–30)	3.77 (4.93; 0–19)
Specific requests for repetition[a]	0.58 (0.9; 0–3)	0
Specific requests for confirmation[b]	4.96 (4.25; 0–18)	2.35 (3.78; 0–16)
Specific requests for specification	1.46 (2.2; 0–10)	1.42 (2.12; 0–9)
Potential requests	7.39 (8.24; 0–34)	4.65 (5.32; 0–24)
Potential requests for elaboration[b]	1.5 (2.55; 0–10)	0.42 (0.9; 0–4)
Potential requests for confirmation	4.54 (5.52; 0–21)	3.31 (3.88; 0–17)
Potential requests for specification	1.35 (1.83; 0–6)	0.92 (1.77; 0–7)

[a]Deaf–hearing higher than controls, $p < 0.01$.
[b]Deaf–hearing higher than controls, $p < 0.05$.

Table 4.6 shows the mean number of non-specific, specific, and potential clarification requests made by the deaf-hearing and control dyads. The deaf–hearing dyads made significantly more non-specific requests for repetition $(t(50) = 3.67, p < 0.01)$ and specific requests for confirmation $(t(50) = 2.36, p < 0.05)$ than the controls. That the deaf–hearing dyads used more repetition requests and more specific confirmation requests than the controls suggests that the use of these types of clarification requests may be viewed as adaptive strategies that are used in situations where communication difficulties arise.

Clarification requests: a comparison between the deaf and hearing members of the deaf–hearing dyads

Table 4.7 shows the frequency and mean number of clarification requests made by the deaf children and their hearing peers. The hearing children made more clarification requests than the deaf, but this difference was not significant. This finding suggests that some of the communication difficulties that occurred within the deaf–hearing dyads went beyond the deaf child's inability to hear their partner's instructions; some of the hearing children had problems with interpreting their deaf partner's instructions.

Table 4.7 Frequency and mean number (SD; range) of clarification requests made by members of the deaf–hearing dyads

	Deaf	Hearing
Frequency	176	246
Mean number	6.77 (5.53; 0–19)	9.46 (13.68; 0–61)

Table 4.8 shows the percentage distribution of non-specific, specific and potential clarification requests made by the deaf children and their hearing peers. A higher proportion of the clarification requests by the deaf children was non-specific compared to that of their hearing partners.

Table 4.8 Percentage distribution of non-specific, specific and potential clarification requests for the members of the deaf–hearing dyads

	Deaf	Hearing
Non-specific	21.59	4.07
Specific	39.78	45.53
Potential	38.63	50.4

Table 4.9 shows the mean number of non-specific, specific, and potential clarification requests made by members of the deaf–hearing dyads. The deaf members made significantly more non-specific requests for repetition than the hearing members ($t(50) = 2.57, p < 0.01$). This finding supports the suggestion of Jeanes, Nienhuys and Rickards (2000) that the increased use of non-specific requests for repetition by deaf children who are communicating orally is an adaptive strategy due to their difficulties with perceiving spoken communication.

There was no significant difference between the number of non-specific, specific and potential requests made by the deaf members. Lloyd's (1999b) literature review suggested that, in comparison to hearing children, deaf children are more likely to use non-specific rather than specific clarification requests. The present results did not support this

Table 4.9 Mean number (SD; range) of non-specific, specific and potential clarification requests made by members of the deaf–hearing dyads

	Deaf	Hearing
Non-specific requests for repetition[a]	1.46 (2.01; 0–7)	0.38 (0.75; 0–2)
Specific requests	2.69 (3.12; 0–13)	4.31 (6.5; 0–30)
Specific requests for repetition	0.31 (0.74; 0–3)	0.27 (0.53; 0–2)
Specific requests for confirmation	1.88 (2.41; 0–9)	3.08 (4.52; 0–18)
Specific requests for specification	0.5 (0.91; 0–3)	0.96 (2.13;0–10)
Potential requests	2.62 (2.73; 0–9)	4.77 (7.75; (0–31)
Potential requests for elaboration	0.5 (1.45; 0–7)	1.0 (2.28; 0–10)
Potential requests for confirmation	1.73 (2.44; 0–8)	2.81 (4.69; 0–21)
Potential requests for specification	0.38 (0.75; 0–3)	0.96 (1.69; 0–6)

[a]Deaf higher than hearing, $p < 0.01$.

finding. These deaf children were as likely to use specific and potential requests as non-specific requests. Although the deaf children made significantly more non-specific requests than their hearing peers, there was no significant difference between the number of specific and potential requests made by the deaf and hearing children. Thus, in this controlled context, deaf children were as likely to use specific and potential requests as they were non-specific requests, and they were as likely to use specific and potential requests as their hearing partners.

Gestures and their use by the deaf–hearing and control dyads

Table 4.10 shows that the deaf–hearing dyads used significantly more supplementary gestures than the controls ($t(50) = 2.70, p < 0.01$). Over half of the deaf–hearing dyads used supplementary gestures, compared to just two of the control dyads. Not surprisingly, there appeared to be a relationship between use of gestures and level of hearing loss (see Table 4.11), with the dyads with children with profound hearing losses using more gestures than those with children with severe hearing losses ($t(24) = 2.65, p < 0.02$). Thus, the control dyads rarely needed to use gestures to convey their messages successfully in this task, but it was evident that some of the deaf–hearing dyads did need to use gestures, particularly some of the dyads with children with profound hearing losses. Frequency of gestures did not correlate with scores of message adequacy ($r = -0.002$) or correct identification of landmarks ($r = 0.1$), but this may have been because the relative simplicity of the task made it easy for some children to perform at ceiling level.

Within the deaf–hearing dyads, the hearing children used more gestures than the deaf (256 as opposed to 147), although this difference was not significant. Some of these hearing children appeared to find it difficult to convey their instructions successfully to their deaf partners without the use of gestures. Although these gestures represented simple concepts (e.g. holding up two fingers when saying 'two doors'), some deaf–hearing dyads appeared to find communication difficult without them.

Table 4.10 Frequency and mean number (SD; range) of gestures by the deaf–hearing and control dyads

	Deaf–hearing	Controls
Frequency of gestures	403	20
No. of dyads who used gestures	15	2
Mean number of gestures[a]	15.5 (27.62; 0–112)	0.77 (3.06; 0–15)

[a]Deaf–hearing higher than controls, $p < 0.01$.

Table 4.11 Mean number (SD; range) of gestures as function of level of hearing loss (severe or profound)

	Severe	Profound
Number of dyads	14	12
Mean number of gestures[a]	3.57 (10.56; 0–32)	29.42 (35.43; 0–112)

[a]Profound higher than severe, $p < 0.02$.

Frequency of gestures, message adequacy, and landmarks correctly identified

Was there a relationship between communicative success in the deaf–hearing dyads and their use of gestures? As mentioned, no significant correlations were found between frequency of gestures and message adequacy or landmarks correctly identified, but Figures 4.6 and 4.7 suggest that the improvement over time in some deaf–hearing dyads may have been related to their use of gestures. Figure 4.6 shows a steady rise in the frequency of gestures between trials 1–4, falling in trials 5 and 6. The fall in the frequency of gestures in trials 5 and 6 was accompanied by a rise in the percentage of adequate messages. Figure 4.7 shows that the percentage of landmarks correctly identified rises steadily between trials 2 and 5. As for adequate messages, the fall in the frequency of gestures in trials 5 and 6 was accompanied by a rise in the percentage of landmarks correctly identified. Consideration of Figures 4.6 and 4.7 suggests an explanation for the improvement over time by some deaf–hearing dyads: it may have taken longer for them to establish mutual understanding in comparison to the controls, perhaps because some of the deaf children relied more heavily on the visual aspects of communication than their partners. For some of the deaf–hearing dyads, some of the moves in the early trials were problematic. Then some children began to realize that their instructions could be conveyed more easily if gestures were used to emphasize the critical information (e.g. holding up two fingers when saying 'two doors'). The increase in the frequency of gestures between trials 1 and 4 may have been instrumental in helping some deaf–hearing dyads to achieve mutual understanding. By trials 5 and 6, they may have essentially mastered the task and therefore been less reliant on the support of gestures than in earlier trials.

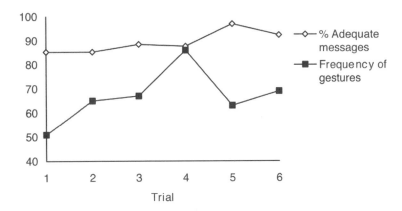

Figure 4.6 Percentage of adequate messages and frequency of gestures by the deaf–hearing dyads as a function of trial.

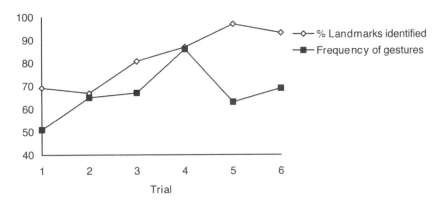

Figure 4.7 Percentage of landmarks identified and frequency of gestures by the deaf–hearing dyads as a function of trial.

Conclusion and directions

The present study has suggested that hearing peers can contribute to the communicative and academic development of deaf children.

Although the deaf–hearing dyads' performance on a route-giving task was initially inferior to that of the hearing–hearing control dyads, it improved in a relatively short time. This finding suggests that collaboration between deaf and hearing pupils can lead to learning and improved communication. It should be noted, however, that the task in the present study was relatively easy for most of the hearing controls, with many of them performing at ceiling level throughout. That the deaf–hearing dyads were performing at a similar level to the controls in the latter trials may have been an artefact of the simple nature of the task, and should not be taken to show that they were then generally communicating as successfully as the control dyads.

As in previous studies, the present findings have suggested that deaf children are more likely to use non-specific requests for repetition than their hearing counterparts. However, as these deaf children used specific and potential requests as often as non-specific requests, and used a similar number of specific and potential requests as their hearing partners, the increased use of non-specific requests may be viewed as an adaptive strategy, which results from the deaf children's difficulties with perceiving spoken communication, rather than as a delay in their acquisition of clarification strategies (see Jeanes, Nienhuys and Rickards, 2000).

In comparison to the controls, the deaf–hearing dyads made significantly more: (1) clarification requests overall; (2) requests for repetition; and (3) specific requests for confirmation. This pattern of results appears to reflect the use of adaptive clarification strategies, resulting from communication difficulties that arose within the deaf–hearing dyads. The use of these strategies is not necessarily related to deafness, however, as they may be typical of other situations in which communication difficulties arise.

Some of the present findings can be interpreted from a Neo-Vygotskian perspective. Though this task did not involve explicit instruction, some deaf–hearing dyads appeared to learn through interacting with each other, and this learning may have been supported by the increased levels of mutual understanding that developed from the use of certain clarification and nonverbal strategies. Though these observed improvements may have been related to practice and task familiarity, practice and familiarity are undoubtedly also related to learning in everyday situations. These findings therefore offer some insight into the types of behaviour that might support collaborative learning between deaf and hearing pupils in other situations. In Neo-Vygotskian terms, it might be argued that the adaptive strategies observed in this study scaffolded learning and improved communication between deaf and hearing children. Thus, the Neo-Vygotskian concept of scaffolding might be particularly important to the future study of interaction between deaf and hearing children. The challenge of future research is to determine the processes that lead to learning and communicative development.

Inside the classroom, peer tutoring and cooperative learning might be used to facilitate the communicative and academic development of deaf children. The present study has illustrated how outcome measures and communicative processes can be studied together, and so it is now suggested that future research examines peer tutoring and cooperative learning between deaf and hearing pupils, and assesses the relationship between learning outcomes and interactive and communicative processes.

The present research has suggested that communication between deaf and hearing pupils is widely varied (see the range of scores in Table 4.3). It is not suggested that every grouping of deaf and hearing pupils will lead to positive outcomes in learning and communicative development. Some hearing peers might be better at scaffolding the communication and learning of deaf children than others, and some deaf children might be better than others at interacting with hearing children. The interactive and communicative processes that scaffold learning and communication between deaf and hearing children need to be determined; these might be different to those that facilitate communication and learning in typically developing children.

- What adaptive strategies are used by deaf and hearing pupils in learning situations, and how do they differ from those used by typically developing children in similar situations?
- Do deaf pupils copy the strategies of their hearing peers or vice versa, or do new strategies evolve as a result of interaction between deaf and hearing pupils?
- Why are some hearing children better at interacting with deaf children than others, and vice versa?
- How does age affect collaborative learning between deaf and hearing pupils?

These are some of the questions that should be addressed in future research. The present study has focused on spoken communication, but the author is not taking a position on the preference or otherwise of an oral approach over signing for deaf children. As discussed in Lloyd, Lieven and Arnold (2001), signing between deaf and hearing children requires further investigation. The present study has shown that some deaf–hearing dyads required gestures to successfully convey their messages in what was a fairly simple task; non-verbal communication between deaf and hearing children should now be investigated in other contexts. This task involved simple concepts, and so it was fairly easy for the participants to incorporate gestures to convey these concepts. It might be much more difficult for deaf and hearing pupils to communicate about topics in the classroom (e.g. a science project). The use of gestures in classrooms, particularly those where Total Communication is used, and hence where the children have exposure to conventional signs, could be a productive focus of future research. Future research should also examine the type of language input that hearing children provide for their deaf peers, and the extent to which deaf children can use the speech styles of their peer groups (see also Lloyd, Lieven and Arnold, 2001).

Acknowledgements

This study was supported by ESRC research studentship number R00429734533. I would like to thank Elena Lieven and Paul Arnold for supervising the project, and Clare Morgans, Vicky Hopwood, Clare Gallaway, Pamela Pitt and Peter Lloyd for their help and advice. A special thank you goes to all the children, teachers and parents who made this research possible.

Chapter 5
Deaf children in hearing classrooms: teacher–pupil talk in secondary schools

VICKY HOPWOOD

Supporting deaf children in the mainstream

At present, most deaf children in the UK are educated in mainstream schools and it is thought that the majority (about 80%) are being educated through spoken language. Deaf children may spend an ever-increasing part of the day in the mainstream classroom and they may also spend some time in small withdrawal groups. In both these situations they receive support from a number of adults. Research conducted in recent years has shown that the trend towards mainstreaming deaf pupils has led to a change in the role of teachers and support staff. Differences have been highlighted in terms of the amount and location of the support provided, the methods used, who provides the support, and in what context. Much of the support provided is effected via spoken language and it is the nature of the deaf child's experience of spoken language that is investigated in this study, within the mainstream class and via other support staff.

The task of the Teacher of the Deaf (ToD) within the mainstream school is very different from that of ToDs in special school contexts (Lynas, Lewis and Hopwood, 1997; Watson and Parsons, 1998). In the latter, the ToD provides the curriculum and promotes language development through direct teaching, whereas in the former the ToD role is to facilitate and support access to the curriculum – the class teacher is ultimately responsible for the content (Lynas, Lewis and Hopwood, 1997). The ToD needs to ensure that classrooms which are not specifically tailored to meet the needs of deaf pupils are nevertheless supportive of language development and pupil access to the curriculum. Their task then is to 'facilitate education rather than directly provide it.

The role thus becomes essentially one of management and support'
(Lynas, Lewis and Hopwood, 1997:42). Nevertheless, this definition of
the function of ToDs in ordinary schools does not dictate the types of
activities employed, which vary as a result of external influences.

Deaf children in mainstream schools receive variable amounts of support (Lynas, 1999a, 1999b). Often they are not supported full-time, so
increasingly the responsibility for instructing them rests with mainstream staff who may not have specialist training or knowledge. Support
offered can vary in location, either in withdrawal groups or units or in-
class. In the study by Lynas (1999a), all the deaf pupils were withdrawn
from the classroom from time to time. Withdrawing pupils from the
mainstream class provides opportunities for enhancing speech and language within a quiet and relaxed environment (Lynas, 1999a). In the
past, the practice of withdrawing deaf pupils for considerable periods
for specialist teaching was common, but increasingly, this practice is
being discouraged (Mittler, 1989). Providing support within the classroom itself, in-class support, is becoming more prevalent (Powers,
1990). According to research (Lynas, 1986; Gregory and Bishop, 1989),
in-class support was far less common 10 years ago.

A variety of personnel are now employed to support deaf pupils.
Aside from ToDs, audiologists and speech and language therapists, var-
iously labelled support staff feature increasingly in the support
structure (Fletcher-Campbell, 1992; Walker, 1993; Roberts and Rickards,
1994; Monkman and Baskind, 1998). Some deaf students are now being
supported by adults with little or no specialist training or knowledge. It
has been argued that to facilitate language development in deaf children, support adults need detailed knowledge (Reich, Hambleton and
Houldin, 1977; Tucker and Powell, 1991).

The nature of the language experience that arises as a result of varying support practices remains relatively unexplored. Hopwood's study
was an attempt to investigate the language input and interaction resulting from a variety of teaching practices used with secondary aged deaf
pupils in mainstream schools.

The acquisition of spoken language and classroom interaction

Language acquisition arises, in part, from interaction between children
and adults. This process proceeds with ease during the early years. For
profoundly deaf children, however, developing spoken language is
likely to be problematic and many are still acquiring their spoken language skills throughout the school years. For this reason an
understanding of deaf children's language environment in school is
important. It is also important because in the current educational

climate the routines of teaching and learning have changed with the growing trend towards inclusion.

The conditions in which infants acquire their first language is within the family, often in one-to-one conversations with adults, and by the time they arrive at school, basic language skills are in place; nevertheless, infants at four years can still find the home–school transition difficult (Geekie and Raban, 1994). Pupils are generally not permitted to initiate turns whenever they wish, as they are in family household conversation (Willes, 1981), and receive fewer opportunities to engage in one-to-one interaction. Their chances to question adults are relatively infrequent when compared to the opportunities presented to them at home.

In school, the teacher dominates and children are expected to answer questions and to respond to requests (Richards and Gallaway, 1994). Teacher questioning tends to be specific in nature and is typically designed to elicit factual recall from pupils. Most teachers desire a specific response to their questions and requests, and in this way a primary purpose of classroom conversation is, amongst other things, a means for checking pupil knowledge, understanding and to manage behaviour, rather than for communicative purposes per se (Stubbs, 1990; Hopwood and Gallaway, 1999). Classroom discourse is characteristically structured so that the teacher initiates the interaction (typically through question forms), the pupil replies and then the teacher evaluates the response (Barnes, 1969). This has been seen as having negative consequences for encouraging pupil dialogue that nourishes language development. In short, as Hopwood and Gallaway (1999; p. 175) write, ' 'teacherese' is not 'motherese', and its functions are more likely to be those of management and control . . . rather than facilitat[ing] language acquisition'.

This is of potentially great consequence for deaf children who are often still acquiring a linguistic system throughout their school years. Deaf children entering school by and large have not reached the same level of linguistic competence as their hearing peers. Provision for further acquisition of language in school therefore becomes of utmost importance (Watson, 1998; Hopwood and Gallaway, 1999). It is thought that just as mother–child interaction impacts on deaf children's language acquisition, so does the language used by teachers and educators.

Wood and Wood (1984) constructed an experiment which found that correlations between teacher style and child loquacity were causal in nature. This suggests that if teachers wish to promote conversational participation by their deaf pupils then is it perhaps best to avoid frequent questioning. Although pupil participation in conversation may not be generally necessary in classroom talk to normal learners, it is often advocated with deaf children as a means for promoting language competence and growth. Easterbrooks (1998) claims that fostering language skills in students means engaging them in conversation. She argues this is a classroom skill that needs to be promoted with hearing impaired pupils because it not only aids communicative development, but also because as the child's age increases so do the demands to engage in lengthy discourse in school.

Classroom interaction with deaf pupils attending ordinary classes is only just beginning to receive systematic attention by research. Much of the evidence in this area comes from studies abroad, most noticeably Spain and America (Saur et al., 1987; Caissie and Wilson, 1995; Miller, 1995; Valero Garcia, 1999). Valero Garcia (1999) observed 15 profoundly deaf students in mainstream primary and secondary schools in Spain interacting with their ordinary class teacher. Valero Garcia found that lower levels of communicative control exerted by the teacher were related first, to the amount of experience and knowledge the ordinary teacher had of working with deaf pupils; second, to higher linguistic capabilities in children; and third, to the 'educative cycle'. Valero Garcia found that the teacher in the primary school devoted more time and 'interactions' to the deaf student than was the case in the secondary school. Valero Garcia argues that this may be due to the 'all-inclusive nature of the learning programme' in the early school years which obliges the teacher to give more individual attention to the students. Valero Garcia's work seems to suggest that the situation of control increases the further the child progresses through schooling.

Miller (1995:29) has argued that one of the best ways to facilitate language development in deaf children is to 'give them opportunities to use their English skills in a purposeful way during the school day'. Although in the normal classroom setup opportunities for deaf children to do this are rare, Miller argues it is possible to find ways of shaping classrooms so that deaf children are encouraged in conversational dialogue. Caissie and Wilson (1995) have suggested that, although deaf children in ordinary classes frequently face communication breakdown during cooperative learning, training in clarification techniques can help (on this topic, see also Chapter 4, this volume.)

In summary, there is a good deal of literature concerning the nature of language in the classroom in general, but practically none which inform on the specific nature of teacher–pupil talk with deaf pupils in the mainstream.

The nature of Hopwood's study

The aims of the study were:

- to understand and evaluate the variation in language input to deaf children in school
- to determine whether the linguistic environment provided by the support ToD or learning support assistant was likely to be facilitative
- to investigate how differing contexts of support (in-class versus withdrawal) affected the language input received by the deaf child.

The subjects were 19 severely or profoundly oral deaf pupils, aged 11–14, who were observed in mainstream secondary school classes in England. They were video- and audio-recorded in varying naturalistic contexts, including:

- withdrawal sessions
- in the mainstream classroom supported by a ToD or support assistant
- in the mainstream classroom without any additional support present.

The language interactions were transcribed and analysed, using a framework designed for the classroom context (Sinclair and Coulthard, 1975; for further details, see Hopwood, 2000). From the variety of exchange structures identified, two are considered here:

- teacher-led question and answer exchanges
- support exchanges.

The IRF exchange

The work of Sinclair and Coulthard (1975) showed that question and answer sequences in the classroom have a definite structure that is typically repeated. This is usually in the form: teacher asks (I), pupil answers (R), the teacher comments (F), and then the sequence starts again.

> Teacher: what are you doing in science at the moment? Initiation (I)
> Child: using keys. Response (R)
> Teacher: you're using keys, that's right. Follow-up (F)
> (Unless stated, all examples are taken from Hopwood, 2000).

As has been corroborated in a number of studies of classroom interaction (Johnson and Griffith, 1986; Nunan, 1987; McCarthy, 1991; Wells, 1993; Cullen, 1998) this IRF communicative exchange structure was common to all data sets in this study. These exchanges were then subjected to fine-grained analysis and it was found that there were subtle but important differences within the IRF structure which may be considered to have differing consequences in terms of language development.

The initiating move

First, differences were identified in terms of the first move in the sequence – the initiating move. This can be exemplified in the extracts shown in Table 5.1. Although all these have the same basic IRF communicative exchange structure, there are differences in terms of the question function.

Table 5.1 TQs, DQs and RQs

Line no.	Speaker	Text	Move	Act
Extract 1 (TQ)				
480	Teacher:	how many little markings have we got in that centimetre?	I	el
481	Child:	ten.	R	rep
482	Teacher:	ten right	F	e
Extract 2 (DQ)				
16	Teacher:	has anybody got anything that they could add to that?	I	el
17	Teacher:	Jennifer.		n
18	Child:	it's like erm if there was a pin and you wanted to see what it's really like xx right inside you can make it so that you can see.	R	rep
19	Teacher:	right.	F	e
Extract 3 (RQ)				
397	TOD:	so how how d'you feel about taking it?	I	el
398	Deaf child:	yes.	R	rep
399	Deaf child:	probably really.		rep
400	Deaf child:	so long as I don't have to do that written <work again> [>].		rep
401	TOD:	<no> [<].	F	ack

F, follow-up; I, initiation; R, response; xx indicates untranscribable talk; < > indicates overlapping talk.

In extract 1, the teacher's question has a known right answer. Such questions were labelled test questions (TQs).

In extract 2, the teacher may have a series of possible responses which she considers appropriate or acceptable but she does not know which of these options will be given. The teacher's question is concerned with getting the pupils to display knowledge of a certain topic. These questions were labelled display questions (DQs).

In extract 3, the question is concerned with the pupil's feelings or opinion. The question is designed to encourage the pupil to talk, to express an opinion or feelings, or to explain thoughts – in other words for genuine communicative purposes. Such questions were labelled real questions (RQs).

TQs serve the function of testing knowledge, an important educational function. However, in terms of language development, use of TQs can be questioned as they do not encourage pupils to talk. Responses are generally minimal. DQs are also used for pedagogic purposes, to get pupils to display their knowledge. The DQs identified in this study seemed to encourage more participation in the child than did the TQs. However, ultimately this depended on the extent of the pupils' knowledge of the subject area. RQs were used for a variety of reasons by different staff. Sometimes they were used with the aim of finding out what the pupil had been doing in school, or what the pupil knew about the topic they were working on. This was more commonly the case when ToDs were working with deaf pupils, when they wanted to know what the child had been doing in school. RQs were seldom used by class teachers to initiate talk about anything other than education. When class teachers did use an RQ to communicate on a non-educational topic, the exchange tended to be very short and quick. However, ToDs within withdrawal situations used the RQ far more. How successfully the RQ promoted conversational exchange however, was found to be linked to the adult's use of the F move.

The prevalence of different question forms was related to different teaching situations. TQ and DQs during IRF exchanges were more a feature of mainstream classroom discourse and withdrawal sessions that were used for the specific purpose of pre- or post-tutoring the deaf child on a curriculum topic. Use of these is to be expected since they serve the important educational function of ensuring the children know and understand the information being taught. RQs during the mainstream classroom were infrequent and tended to be used as a means to find out whether the pupils had prior experience of the topic. Non-education-related RQs were even more infrequent during mainstream classroom discourse and where they were used the talk did not continue over a number of exchanges. Only in withdrawal situations however, were RQs used to promote more lengthy communicative exchange on non-educational topics. These tended to feature more prominently at either the beginning or the end of the session.

The follow-up move

Second, differences were identified in terms of the third move in the sequence – the follow-up move. The follow-up move was used in a variety of ways. For instance, it was used to evaluate whether the response given was correct (Extract 4 in Table 5.2).

Table 5.2 Use of the follow-up move

Line no.	Speaker	Text	Move	Act
Extract 4				
23	Teacher:	what do we mean by invertebrates?	I	el
24	Child:	it means like they've got no backbone.	R	rep
25	Teacher:	right.	F	e
Extract 5				
50	Teacher:	what else does it do?	I	el
51	Child:	holds the ribs.	R	rep
52	Teacher:	right it holds the ribs.	F	e

The follow-up move was also used both to evaluate and to echo a pupil response. In this way the follow-up serves a dual function – to signal that the reply given was correct, and to offer a means of ensuring the rest of the class has heard what the pupil said so that the interaction can continue with everybody following it (Extract 5 in Table 5.2).

There were other instances when the feedback given in the follow-up move was used in a slightly different way. For example, the follow-up move was used not only to signal to the pupil whether the response given was right or wrong but whether the language used was correct or appropriate. This involved recasting the child's utterance in a revised or expanded form. There were some instances where the adult's feedback was in the form of a grammatical recast. However, there were other instances where the feedback involved vocabulary correction or presentation of the child's utterance in the form of an extended sentence. In this way, any feedback which offered 'possible information' to the child in terms of the language they used (because it involved correcting the child's grammar, or vocabulary, or extending their response), was labelled corrective feedback (Saxton and Gallaway, 1998). Examples are given in Table 5.3.

Table 5.3 Corrective feedback

Line no.	Speaker	Text	Move	Act
Extract 6				
100	TOD:	what does food that's good for you make you do and make you feel like?	I	el
101	Deaf child:	it makes you give energy.	R	rep
102	TOD:	yes it gives you lots of energy.	F	e
Extract 7				
385	TOD:	do you know what focus means?	I	el
386	Deaf child:	erm move it up and down.	R	rep
387	TOD:	it means wind it up and down but what does it mean if it's in focus?	F Ib	e el

A further distinction in the nature of the follow-up move was also found. In extract 8 (Table 5.4) the follow-up move is sub-classified as an 'acknowledge act' (Sinclair and Coulthard, 1975). The function of an acknowledge act according to Sinclair and Coulthard is to show that the initiation has been understood. In the data transcribed in this study the acknowledge act was frequently used during IRF exchange structures when the initiating move was realized by a real question (RQ). This then prompted the pupil to make further contribution to the talk.

The follow-up move can therefore be used in different ways. With the exception of single-word follow-ups (e.g. 'yes'), these can be considered to have a number of positive consequences. First, follow-up can be used as a means of ensuring the pupils are following the lesson and second, it can be used to encourage deaf children to converse further. Use of follow-up strategies in this way was generally a feature of interaction

Table 5.4 An acknowledge act

Line no.	Speaker	Text	Move	Act
Extract 8				
291	TOD:	with the before we do the science you know the did your mum talk to you about the food technology?		
292	TOD:	the NVQ exam?	I	el
293	Deaf child:	erm	rep	R
294	Deaf child:	um		
295	Deaf child:	she said that		
	Deaf child:	I didn't have to do it again if I didn't I don't want to		
296	TOD:	mmm	F	ack

between deaf pupils and ToDs in the withdrawal situation, and was also a strategy used by both class teachers and support personnel.

Implications of the IRF structure: effective or non-effective?

> If there is one finding on which students of classroom discourse are agreed, it must be the ubiquity of the three-part exchange structure . . . (Wells, 1993:1).

The IRF exchange sequence has been commonly identified in classroom discourse as the predominant manner in which the teacher converses in school (Wells, 1993). In seeking to evaluate this structure in terms of its educational significance and effect on language and communication, however, the IRF structure has generated much discussion and divergences of opinion. Some have argued that use of the IRF exchange structure in classroom discourse has negative implications both as an educational device and in terms of language development (Nunan, 1987; Thornbury, 1996). Others would plead conversely, arguing that the IRF exchange is effective as an educational tool and can be viewed to have a more positive relationship to language development (Seedhouse, 1996; Cullen, 1998).

The notion that the IRF exchange structure has negative implications is based on the view that as it is the teacher who provides both the initiating and the follow-up move, the discourse is one-sided and controlled by the teacher. It has been further argued that because of this the communication is not 'genuine' or 'natural' (Seedhouse, 1996). Based on findings from language interaction research, it has been suggested that using language which closely parallels that used in the home situation best facilitates language development in the classroom. Classroom interaction following the IRF structure is not believed by some to do this. In 'genuine' or 'natural' conversation all communicators have an equal right to speak, to initiate dialogue and to respond when they consider it appropriate (Musselman and Hambleton, 1990). By contrast, talk in school is dominated by the teacher. It is the teacher who decides who will talk and when, who chooses the topic of interaction and who controls the talk through questioning (Musselman and Hambleton, 1990). Therefore, because the IRF exchange results in an unequal allotment of power in terms of the talk used, it has been seen to be incompatible with 'natural' or 'communicative' language teaching (Dinsmore, 1985). Furthermore, the questions used have similarly been criticized. Generally a division has been made in terms of whether the question used is an RQ (to which the teacher does not know the answer) or a DQ (which functions to allow pupils to display knowledge) (Thornbury, 1996). Teachers have been accused of using too many questions, especially those for which the teacher already knows the answer (Wood, 1992). DQs have been seen to be non-communicative (Nunan, 1987). This is again based on contrasting 'natural' communication, where a high degree of RQs are used, with classroom discourse, where questions tend to be largely of the DQ variety.

It has also been argued that if teachers want to know what pupils think, and if they want to encourage pupil initiation, then they should use talk in the classroom which is less controlling (Wood, 1992). This arguably is considered better in educational terms, because learning is facilitated by pupils talking their ideas through and thinking things for themselves. The IRF exchange structure may therefore be viewed in negative terms both educationally and linguistically because it results in talk which is dominated by the teacher, talk which is 'unnatural', talk which does not encourage pupil participation and use of DQs which have the same negative connotations.

However, the IRF exchange structure can be viewed in a more positive light when it is viewed in terms of its educational function. In the classroom the IRF sequence is an effective means of monitoring pupil knowledge and comprehension (Mercer, 1992; Cullen, 1998). When examining classroom discourse in mainstream schools in relation to deaf learners, we cannot ignore the fact that the classroom lessons are not essentially designed for the deaf children who attend them. We cannot solely evaluate the talk used in relation to how it promotes or discourages language acquisition. Classrooms are used first and foremost for pedagogic purposes and this needs to be taken into account when evaluating the interaction that takes place. To view the impact of the IRF exchange purely in terms of its relationship to language development and to attempt to inform teacher practice based on an evaluation of this, would be to ignore the fundamental purpose of the classroom. The TQs and DQs used in this study did seem to be effective as an educational device.

Nevertheless, if we do evaluate the IRF exchange and the questions used in the school classroom in terms of their implications for language development we could argue that the relationship between the two is far more complex than the 'negative' viewpoint would have us believe. The idea that talk outside the classroom is more 'natural', 'genuine' or 'communicative' than talk within the classroom can be challenged. The notion that classrooms are uncommunicative is based on the belief that IRF sequences and use of display questions, although predominant in classroom discourse, are rarely a feature in language outside the classroom. Seedhouse (1996) has argued that although IRF sequences are not salient in adult-to-adult talk, they are a very noticeable feature in parent–child interaction, and the same applies to DQs. The IRF exchange has also been identified in interaction between deaf children and their mothers (Plapinger and Kretschmer, 1991). It could be argued, therefore, that to see classroom talk and use of the IRF exchange negatively because it results in talk that is non-communicative and not reflective of talk used outside the classroom is a misconception. Although previous writers (Seedhouse, 1996; Cullen, 1998) have suggested this, they have failed to identify precisely how the follow-up move can be seen as beneficial. This study has found that when the follow-up move is used to expand and recast utterances it can be seen to have positive links to language development.

With regard to question use, it has generally been argued that RQs are 'better' than DQs but that DQs, although negative in terms of language development, do have a positive function in the classroom (Seedhouse, 1996; Cullen, 1998). By refining the definition of questions and viewing these in the categories of TQ, DQ and RQ, this study has shown that the relationship of these in terms of conversational participation is complex. In particular use of DQs can elicit participation from the child and not simply in terms of knowledge but in terms of how they view and think about an educational concept. Similarly, there is some difficulty in evaluating the use of RQs. Some RQs are not simply used to generate communication and talk but also serve an educational purpose of finding out what experience the child has of a certain area. This may therefore not encourage lengthy pupil contributions. In part, positive and negative aspects of the questions used relate to what happens in the follow-up move. Previous research, although extremely influential in informing on the relationship between teacher talk and language development in the deaf (Wood et al, 1986), focused only on the question asked and the response given. This study has shown how attention to the next move, the follow-up, is important in determining the effectiveness or non-effectiveness of questioning on language development.

This study has demonstrated that the IRF exchange and its relationship to education and language development is a complex one. The merits of the structure seem to be related to how and why it is used. Perhaps then we should not be calling for its use to be withdrawn but concentrating on a refinement of its description. The findings of this study suggest that this means varying how both the initiating and follow-up moves are used, a finding which has been similarly suggested in previous literature (Wells, 1993; Kretschmer and Kretschmer, 1995).

Support exchange

Support exchanges, as they were identified in this study, are those in which there is more than one adult inputting to the deaf child within a mainstream lesson. As there was more than one adult inputting talk to the deaf child, it was extremely difficult to determine the structural sequence of these exchanges. This is due to the fact that ultimately two 'conversations' were, in effect, taking place. In these exchanges the talk of the class teacher to the whole class, of which the deaf child was a part, was under consideration, together with the talk of the support adult to the deaf pupil. In these situations the class teacher's talk may follow a particular exchange structure. The talk of the supporting adult may be used to fit in with the exchange structure of the class teacher or may have an entirely different structure of its own. In cases where a support exchange was occurring, the researcher separated out the talk of the class teacher and that of the support adult. The structural sequences were first analysed separately. They were then put back together to see how this affected the exchange. This enabled the researcher to consider how, or if, the talk of the support adult related to that of the class teacher. It also enabled the researcher to make a detailed consideration of the talk when there was a great deal of over-lap, in other words, when there were two people inputting to the deaf pupil at once. This may be labelled as co-tutoring (Table 5.5).

By separating out the talk of the class teacher we can see that the class teacher recycles the original question until he receives the desired response.

The second stage is to separate out the talk of the support adult, in this case a ToD, to see if her talk gives an identifiable exchange structure.

The talk of the ToD in Table 5.6 does not fit in with a particular exchange structure (as defined by Sinclair and Coulthard, 1975) and is thus part of a bigger support exchange (Hopwood, 2000). Indeed the talk of the ToD in this case is being used to fit in with, or reinforce, the talk of the class teacher. This becomes clear just by looking at the ToD's first initiation. She says 'you know that'. If the deaf pupils had not already been given the input from the class teacher then they would have no idea what the 'that' is referring to. The ToD gives the hearing impaired pupils a second chance to hear the class teacher's original question in line 46, when she repeats the teacher's question. However, the point is that her opening move would not have made sense without

Table 5.5 The Support Exchange.
Note: sequences that overlap each other are indicated by a number.

Line no.	Speaker	Text
Extract 9a		
38	Teacher:	can anybody tell me what the formula for pressure is?
39	TOD:	you know that
40	Teacher:	pressure equals
41	Teacher:	Jeremy
42	Child 1:	yes
43	Teacher:	what's the formula for pressure?
44	Teacher:	<pressure equals> [>1]
45	TOD:	<you know that> [<1]
46	TOD:	<what's the formula for pressure> [>2]?
47	Teacher:	<have a look in the book> [<2]
48	Child 1:	area
49	Child 2:	area divided by
50	Teacher:	shush
51	Teacher:	hands up if you know
52	TOD:	stick your hands up
53	Teacher:	hands up if you think you know
54	Comment:	LUC has her hand up
55	Teacher:	Lucy
56	Teacher:	pressure
57	Deaf child:	force divided by area
58	Teacher:	that's it, force divided by area

Table 5.6 The extracted talk of the teacher of the deaf

Line no.	Speaker	Text	Move	Act
Extract 9b				
39	TOD:	You know that.	I	cue
45	TOD:	<you know that> [<1].	I	cue
46	TOD:	<what's the formula for pressure> [>2]?	I	el
52	TOD:	Stick your hands up		d
54	Comment:	Deaf child puts her hand up		

the class teacher's move having been given first. In this extract the ToD's talk is supplementary but linked to the talk of the class teacher. The ToD is trying to make sure the deaf pupils are taking part in the talk of the class lesson. She encourages them to do this through a series of cues and directing acts, telling the deaf pupils they do know the answer to the class teacher's question and should put their hands up. She also repeats the class teacher's question for them in a simpler form. The supplementary contributions of the ToD seem to have been effective, as it is one of the deaf pupils who provides the answer to the class teacher's original question in line 57.

This example shows one way in which additional adults use support exchanges when offering support in-class in mainstream lessons. This may be determined as contributing to, or providing supplementary talk to, the exchange sequence used by the class teacher. The supplementary talk is used to assist or encourage the deaf pupils in answering a question. This can be an effective means of ensuring the deaf pupils are taking part in and understanding the class teacher's talk in the mainstream class lesson.

However, support exchanges of this type were not always found to be as successful as the one given here. Instances were identified in which the talk of the ToD seemed, on the one hand, to link in with the talk of the class teacher but on the other, seemed to have some structure of its own. It was not entirely clear in these instances whether the talk of the ToD was matched to that of the class teacher or whether it had an agenda of its own. Exchanges of this type did not appear to be as successful as that given above for a number of reasons. First, much of the talk of the ToD overlapped with that of the class teacher. Second, the ToD seemed to switch between taking part in the exchange of the class teacher and pursuing one of her own. This may cause the deaf pupils some difficulty as they may be unsure who they are supposed to be listening to. This is exacerbated by the fact that, by virtue of their impairment, it is very difficult for the deaf pupils to tune in and pick out different parts of different conversations simultaneously. In this way the ToD may well have distracted from the class exchange sequence occurring.

This suggests that if supporting adults are going to contribute to the talk of the class lesson simultaneously with the class teacher then they have to do so sensitively. This means signposting to the deaf pupils where the talk is going and whether, or how, it is to be considered in association with the talk of the class teacher.

Other forms of support exchange, although providing talk to supplement information given by the class teacher, did not seem to be connected with the exchange the class teacher was pursuing at the time. This is examined in extract 10 (Table 5.7).

In this extract, the class teacher is giving a lengthy answer to an initiation from one of the hearing pupils in the class. Towards the end of the extract, the ToD starts to talk simultaneously to the deaf pupil she is supporting. Much of the initial talk has been included in this extract to provide background and contextual detail.

If we look at the talk of the ToD which commences in line 428, we can see that her exchange seems to be separate and not linked with the exchange sequence of the class teacher.

As the talk of the ToD is overlapping with that of the class teacher this exchange has been identified as part of a support exchange. However, when considered separately, it would appear that the exchange has a

Table 5.7 How the teacher of the deaf can reinforce areas of misunderstanding

Line no.	Speaker	Text	Move	Act
Extract 10a				
408	Child:	Right sir you know like being up in space like the moon yes?	I	el
409	Child:	Why aren't they up in the sea?		el
410	Teacher:	Well in fact it's a very good question that Andrew	R	rep
411	Teacher:	And the answer is that because (basically) [>1]	R	rep
412	Child:	<xx xx> [<1]	Uncodable	
413	Teacher:	I'll tell you two things actually	R	i
414	Teacher:	number one is that		i
415	Teacher:	when I was a bit older than you but not very much when I was around about twenty		i
416	Teacher:	the Russians		i
417	Teacher:	in nineteen fifty seven the Russians got s the first satellite into space		i
418	Teacher:	and the Americans had always thought that they were the best and the biggest		i
419	Comment:	background chatter		
420	Teacher:	and then in nineteen sixty one the Russians got the first man into space		i
421	Teacher:	may have been nineteen fifty nine actually		i
422	Child:	man or xx?	I	el
423	Teacher:	the first man into space	I	l
424	Child:	xx someat	I	el
425	Teacher:	shut up listen and let me finish.	R	d
426	Teacher:	<and some of the Americans decided no I've got that wrong sorry I've got that wrong altogether> [>1]	R	i
427	Teacher:	no that's right yes the the America	R	i
428	TOD:	<do you understand what he was saying before about this> [<1]?	I	el
429	Comment:	the deaf pupil shakes his head	R nv	rea
430	TOD:	<before he thought they always thought things couldn't live if it was too hot or too cold> [>2]	I	com
431	TOD:	<but now now we have found out that there are some things that can live in very hot conditions and very cold conditions> [>2]	I	i
432	TOD:	<so maybe that means that there could be things living on other planets> [>2]	I	
433	Teacher:	<in nineteen fifty I think it was nineteen fifty nine the Americans the the Russians got the first man into space on the satellite> [<2]	R	
Extract 10b				
428	TOD:	<do you understand what he was saying before about this> [>1] ?	I	el
429	Comment:	the deaf pupil shakes his head.	R nv	rea
430	TOD:	<before he thought they always thought things couldn't live if it was too hot or too cold> [>1].	I	com
431	TOD:	<but now now we have found out that there are some things that can live in very hot conditions and very cold conditions> [>1].	I	i
432	TOD:	<so maybe that means that there could be things living on other planets> [>1].	I	

structure of its own. The talk of the ToD within this support exchange seems to be being used as a check. The ToD uses her initiating move in line 428 to check that the deaf pupil understands what has already been talked about in the course of the lesson. The deaf pupil shakes his head. The ToD then uses her talk to inform the deaf pupil and to recap the information that the class teacher has already given.

In this support exchange, then, the talk of the ToD is being used to supplement the talk of the class teacher but is being used to supplement a sequence of talk that occurred earlier in the lesson. In the exchange pursued in this extract the class teacher is giving lots of information based on a pupil elicit. The ToD seems to consider the detail given by the class teacher as not central to the main aim of the lesson. Therefore, she uses this as an opportunity to check that the deaf pupil has followed the lesson so far and as an opportunity to reinforce areas of misunderstanding.

Support exchanges were therefore used as a means for the support adult to supplement the talk given by the class teacher. As has been demonstrated, this may be used in conjunction with a currently occurring exchange sequence or to supplant it. Support exchanges generally featured when a ToD was providing in-class support rather than a support assistant, who tended to remain quiet. Reinforcement of the lesson topic was generally conducted towards the end of the lesson when the children were engaged in their work. No conclusions can be made with regard to this, however, as it could well be that the types of lessons, which were transcribed while a support assistant was present, did not call for exchanges of this type. The success of the support exchange in supporting learning seems variable and open to different interpretations. Some exchange sequences seemed to enhance the participation and understanding of the deaf pupils in the lesson, but the success of others was more indeterminate. Certainly it could be argued that it is beneficial to use periods when the class teacher seems to be engaged in exchanges that are not central to the lesson aim to reinforce work already presented.

Conclusions

A fine-grained analysis of question and answer sequences in mainstream classrooms reveals a complex situation. It would be valuable to understand how far the still continuing spoken language development of deaf children in secondary school classrooms is being helped or hindered by the language experiences, and in particular, teacher–pupil exchanges. This study has defined a useful analytical framework, which though widely used, had hitherto not been applied to the specific context of deaf children in the mainstream and has also focused on some exchanges which may be interpreted as language-facilitative. Much more future investigation is needed, including spoken and signed support and an assessment of the wider educational context.

Acknowledgements

This study was supported by the ESRC, research studentship number R0042963065. I would like to thank Clare Gallaway and Wendy Lynas for supervising the project, and Dan Mansfield and Julian Lloyd for their help and advice. A special thank you goes to all the children, teachers and parents who made this research possible.

PART II
FOCUSING ON PROGRESS AND ATTAINMENT

Commentary

ALYS YOUNG AND CLARE GALLAWAY

The educational attainment of deaf children remains an ongoing concern for parents and professionals alike. Also, for many deaf adults reviewing their childhood educational experiences, the conclusion is all too often one of not having reached their full potential in school. In the UK over the last 20 years there have been many and far-reaching changes in the education offered to deaf children; nonetheless research here into their attainments during that period has been quite limited, with much more relevant research being carried out in the US (Powers, 1998). The chapters in this section address three core priorities in researching deaf children's educational achievement and experience:

- The need for reliable measures of deaf children's actual attainment in key subjects and over time if the effectiveness of educational practice is to be evaluated and standards raised.
- The importance of addressing the particular preferences, styles and challenges of deaf learners in order to refine the processes of teaching and learning.
- The significance of viewing academic progress within a wider developmental context in which other influences on deaf children's development affect their educational attainment.

Tate and colleagues (Chapter 6) address the core issue of measuring actual attainment in key subject areas. As well as presenting some of the most current data available for primary-aged children in the UK, they also outline in detail the methodological challenges involved in ensuring that deaf children are tested fairly by means that do not disadvantage them. Their attention both to culturally reduced assessments of ability, and to the standardization of test instructions in several languages and modalities, significantly increases the validity of their

92

findings. Powers has noted that, in the search for increasing school effectiveness, the regular monitoring of deaf pupils' attainments would be a first step, and that 'much more comprehensive information is needed in order to provide benchmarks for parents, educators and policy-makers ' (Powers, 1998:234). This chapter reports work that moves significantly towards these goals.

Rather than end point attainment, Swanwick (Chapter 7) considers the processes of educational achievement through a close focus on child learning strategies and styles – in this case in relation to the literacy development of sign bilingual children. Once again, it is the very particular demands of the research question that drive methodological innovation. A means was required of eliciting written English data from children that could provide a window into the influence of both the BSL and spoken language abilities of the children on their emerging literacy.

For Hindley (Chapter 8), educational attainment is fundamentally linked to the social and emotional functioning of deaf children. Such development is regarded as a core component in deaf children achieving their academic potential. He reviews the evidence for the difficulties many deaf children experience in developing age appropriate problem-solving strategies, social skills and emotionally sophisticated responses. The extent to which a specialized curriculum in school for promoting social and emotional development is also effective in influencing child behaviour at home is also considered.

Taken together, these three chapters are indicative of the different varieties of research evidence required for developing a better understanding of what influences deaf children's educational progress. Their perspectives in many ways mirror those of the children themselves. For them school will inevitably be about achieving particular measurable academic outcomes. But it is also on a day-to-day basis about how to learn in a linguistically complex environment, and what the rest of their experience of life and relationships might have to do with their engagement with education.

Chapter 6
Developing a picture of attainments and progress of deaf pupils in primary schools

GRANVILLE TATE, CHRISTINE MERRELL AND PETER TYMMS

This chapter focuses on primary schools where little is known of the overall educational achievements of deaf and hearing-impaired children. Conrad conducted the last major study (Conrad, 1979). More recently Powers, Gregory and Thoutenhoofd (1998) reviewed over 300 studies. The review enabled them to state:

> Studies consistently report a delay of 2 to 3.5 years of deaf pupils [mathematical abilities] compared with hearing pupils. It is important to note that this is not as great as the delay observed in general in reading, which ranges from 3 to about 7 years. (Powers, Gregory and Thoutenhoofd 1998:77–78).

It can be noted that the word 'delay' is often used in the literature. From a value-added perspective, a pupil's progress is what they can be expected to achieve from what they already have attained. The progress of a pupil may be more, the same or less than predicted but is lost in a comparison without context. The findings of these studies, important as they are in themselves, do not tell us how pupils were progressing year on year. They do not usually take into account the knowledge and language development of the pupil when they started school. The Conclusion and Recommendations section of the report by Powers et al states:

> While there is a significant amount of data, and approximately 300 studies have been consulted, it has been difficult to arrive at an overall perspective on achievement. [. . .] The lack of a longitudinal element to most research [. . .] is particularly significant. A further problem has been the

availability of appropriate tests and procedures for test administration, in general, and for specific groups such as pupils in sign-bilingual approaches.' (Powers, Gregory and Thoutenhoofd, 1998:175).

The DEMAQS[1] project, based in the Curriculum Evaluation and Management (CEM) Centre, University of Durham, aims to put in place some of these missing elements and thereby develop standardized, consistent assessments of deaf children's educational progress.

A small percentage of children with a hearing loss use British Sign Language (BSL) as their first or preferred language. Translation of instructions, procedures and individual questions (administration) are therefore one important aim of the CEM Centre's research.

The project was established to develop a monitoring system to track the attainments, attitudes and relative progress (value-added) of deaf and hearing-impaired children in the UK. It is endorsed by the Education Research Consortium of Deaf Organizations.[2]

The focus of the project has been on developing guidance for the administration of assessments using spoken English, BSL or a combination of spoken English with signs. Deaf and hearing-impaired pupils' progress is monitored using similar indicators to those used to monitor the progress of non-deaf pupils. The assessments in question are On-Entry Baseline, Year 2 and Year 6. These assessments were originally developed for the Performance Indicators in Primary Schools (Tymms, 1999) (PIPS) project and are coordinated by the CEM Centre.

The assessments

The PIPS On-Entry Baseline is administered in the pupil's first term at school and repeated in the final term. It assesses early maths, early reading, English vocabulary and phonics. The latter is optional for deaf pupils. The Year 2 and Year 6 PIPS assessments include assessments of English vocabulary, a culture-reduced measure of cognitive abilities and an assessment of how pupils feel about school, maths and reading. Subject assessments of reading (English), mathematics and, at Year 6, science are included. Maths and science are assessments of subject knowledge and understanding. These are not necessarily tied to knowledge of English.

---

[1] DEMAQS is a collaborative project involving five universities (which form the acronym) from across the UK: Durham, Edinburgh, Manchester, Queens – Belfast and Swansea.

[2] Consortium members are as follows: BATOD (British Association of Teachers of the Deaf), BDA (British Deaf Association), DELTA (Deaf Education Through Listening and Talking), LASER (Language of Sign as an Educational Resource), NATED (National Association for Tertiary Education for Deaf People), NDCS (National Deaf Children's Society), RNID (Royal National Institute for Deaf People).

Assessment and cultural effects

PIPS assessments can be thought of as containing sections and items on a continuum from culturally reduced to high cultural effects. Culturally reduced sections or questions are ones with minimal language content. Higher cultural effects on responses can be expected with test items with higher language content.

The Problems of Position (POP) sections of Year 2 and Year 6 assessments require pupils to join together dots in the right-hand box to form a pattern that matches a model given in the left-hand box (see Moseley, 1976). The initial explanation is accompanied by visual modelling of how to respond and by checking that pupils have understood what they need to do. It is a culturally reduced assessment of cognitive ability. Once the pupil understands what to do, any number of test items of the same type can be given. Conrad (1979) used a similarly culture reduced measure: Raven's Progressive Matrices. His findings indicated that profoundly deaf children had no less abstract or spatial reasoning ability than those who had less hearing loss.

Other sections or particular questions have high cultural effects: the question understanding or the response is embedded in language. The English vocabulary and reading sections are the most highly culturally embedded. Other questions or sections may fall somewhere in between. The mathematics question printed in symbols '5 + 3 = ?' does not involve understanding English, Greek or BSL but it can be asked in English, Greek or BSL. Or the pupil can simply be asked to look at the symbols and answer (as some of the questions do). Many of the maths and science questions have high cultural effects as the knowledge or concepts they attempt to elicit are embedded in language. In terms of sign language users, this is controlled for by the translations. In terms of children educated via spoken English, this is controlled for by other appropriate adaptations in the administration. The questions in the section asking about pupil attitudes to school and subjects may be asked in any language. They are designed to elicit attitudes to these areas.

Knowledge of concepts learned in school subjects is usually assessed in the language that the learners are taught in. For the majority of pupils with a hearing loss this is the case. However for some pupils – the ones whose teachers use BSL – this has usually not been the case. Undoubtedly some pupils learn most of what they know in school because the teachers use BSL or a combination of spoken English with signs. These children's achievements in the mathematics or science syllabuses may be assessed using the PIPS translations.

Academic achievement: language use and hearing loss

The usual way, the historical way, of looking at deaf children's education has its roots in a medical perspective – a deficiency in hearing. This deficiency is then graded in terms of its severity. Four standardized grades of severity are recognized: 'mild', 'moderate', 'severe' and 'profound'. A more neutral term that has also come to be used is levels of 'hearing loss' rather than 'severity'. Educational attainments are then put alongside the hearing loss grading.

Research by linguists over the last 35 years into the nature of sign languages has gone hand in hand with moves to accepting and valuing their use in education. The development of a philosophy of 'Total Communication' was a reflection of this. The use of English (or any other language) and school learning is viewed more from how it can be communicated and barriers to communication. This move toward accepting sign languages in education around the world has, in the last decade especially, led to the development of sign-bilingual education policies (see Pickersgill, 1998).

By asking teachers to indicate their 'teacher presentation' from the three options 'spoken English only', 'BSL', 'SSE/sign system' we have developed an additional perspective from which to view educational attainments and progress. 'Teacher presentation' is used as a reflection of pupil language preferences. The term 'SSE/sign system' is a category to include those teachers who use spoken English whenever they use visual-gestural language. It is an inclusive term for highly 'English-influenced' signing. Instead of only using a hearing loss perspective on assessment we have, in a sense, mixed all the children together into one group (although the whole group is still defined by 'hearing loss') and divided it by 'teacher presentation'.

Teachers' and pupils' language use

We can gain some insight into the relationship between language use and hearing loss by recording 'teacher presentation' for assessments. Figures 6.1 and 6.2 show the self-reported mode of teacher presentation to Year 2 and Year 6 pupils (see Figures 6.14 and 6.15 below for more details of the sample). The pupils in the assessments shown by the graphs in Figures 6.1 and 6.2 were not chosen as random samples. We therefore cannot be sure they accurately represent percentages of pupils in mainstream schools with different hearing loss, or our three categories of teacher presentation, or percentages of pupil preferences for spoken or sign language. Even so, they do contain some useful information and the similarity of the two graphs encourages the view that the results may be generalizable. Extrapolating from Figures 6.1 and 6.2, and assuming that the assessment presentation is the regular teaching approach, teachers use 'spoken English only' to teach most, if not all, children with a 'mild' or 'moderate' hearing loss in mainstream schools. Teachers using either BSL or SSE/sign system teach about 81% of pupils with 'profound' hearing loss and between 20% and 37% of 'severe' pupils. Of course, the graphs do not indicate the effects of school/ service policies on language use by teachers.

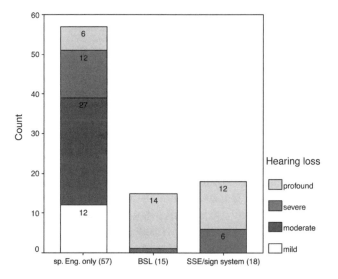

Figure 6.1 Teacher presentation (Year 2).

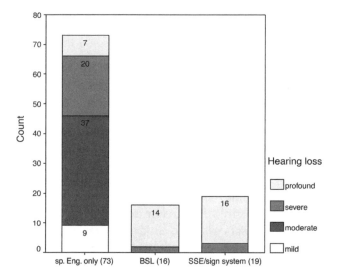

Figure 6.2 Teacher presentation (Year 6).

Teacher guidance: written guidance and BSL guidance (including translation of subject assessments)

Standard ways of presenting instructions and asking questions are required for an assessment to be reliable. Written guidance is provided for presentation with the specific needs of deaf and hearing-impaired pupils considered. Many children with mild and moderate hearing loss will take the PIPS assessments with hearing children and the mainstream teacher. For the teachers of pupils who have visual language preferences, guidance is also provided in BSL that includes translations of individual questions. Without this, teachers would need to create their own and inevitably translate with different versions. Woll (1998) points out:

> One of the main issues in assessing child BSL is the lack of appropriate assessors. Even within bilingual programmes, there is often no individual with bilingual skills: hearing staff may have limited knowledge of BSL and deaf staff may have limited knowledge of English, and neither of these groups may have had any training either in the linguistics of BSL or in the acquisition of BSL. On occasion, language assessments are undertaken by professionals who do not know BSL or who have limited experience of deaf children. Sometimes interpreters are used, which is always unsatisfactory. (Woll, 1998: 67)

The model questions also guide teachers using SSE/sign systems, where visual information that accompanies the spoken English of the teacher may compromise the question being asked: vocabulary signs still need to be the ones used in the BSL question models. Teachers are also guided as to when to use finger-spelling.

The BSL translation of the questions creates a transformed 'frozen' form of the question in BSL and creates a model for standardized presentation to all pupils. As such, this acts as a standard in the way written English models the questions for teachers using only spoken English with a child. Even when interpreters present assessments they still need to follow the guidance and templates of signed questions. To illustrate the point let us consider two questions from the PIPS On-Entry Baseline Assessment (4/5 year olds).

Which bottle will hold the most water?

Which bottle will hold the least water?

The questions assess a level of understanding of the language (in this case English) that is the manifestation of an underlying mathematical concept. The translation must also assess a level of understanding of the language (in this case BSL) as well as the mathematical concept: the language and the mathematical reasoning come as one. Without the guidance, teachers regularly using spoken English with visual support (SSE or a signing system) could decide to use signs or gestures that visually make redundant the assessment of the language plus the concept: a borrowed sign or gesture that is visually motivated by comparative size and volume might be used. This would not produce an accurate assessment of the child's knowledge of the concept, or of English. Teachers regularly using BSL with a child may also use the same strategy. Again, this would not produce a standardized assessment of the child's knowledge of the concept or of BSL. Teachers who regularly use spoken English with a child and at the same time use gestures or signs are using a teaching method designed to aid understanding of English. The methods teachers use in classrooms are not an issue for the assessment. Assessment questions are designed to gather reliable data, and this involves developing questions with a specific aim, which entails standard ways of presentation. Readers are referred to Supalla (1990–91) for research questions concerning whether a language in the spoken modality can be successfully incorporated into a signed modality.

Teachers who wish to administer the assessment using SSE or a signing system will find the BSL models of the questions necessary to the extent that the signing relies on BSL for its sign vocabulary and as a guide to when (or when not) to use finger-spelling to represent English vocabulary. The questions signed in BSL are adaptations that transform the original into a form that can assess the child's knowledge of maths or science concepts (Tate, Collins and Tymms, 2001). The BSL translations of PIPS subject assessments were produced in collaboration with staff of a sign-bilingual service. Other schools and services have also contributed to the process. This has included Deaf, native users of BSL. The teachers were experienced in teaching these subjects to pupils whose preferred language is BSL.

Monitoring achievements of deaf and hearing-impaired pupils from start of reception to Year 2

A large cohort of children with a range of hearing loss (none, mild, moderate, severe or profound) was assessed at the start of reception and end of reception (reported in Tymms et al., 2000). The analysis was constructed on a restricted number of sections taken from the full reception assessment. It demonstrated how prediction of academic achievement of young children with all ranges of hearing loss is possible. Of approximately 112 000 children assessed in reception, 987 had a hearing loss (0.88%). Approximately 52 000 children were assessed in Year 2 and of these approximately 35 000 were assessed for maths and reading. Of the 987 children with a hearing loss assessed in reception, 168 were included in the Year 2 sample. The scores for the whole cohort from each assessment point were normalized, and given a mean of 50 and standard deviation of 10. This enabled comparisons over time to be made for maths and reading. Table 6.1 gives details of the sample of pupils with a hearing loss.

Table 6.1 Pupils with a hearing loss assessed in reception and Year 2 (maths and reading)

Hearing loss	Number of children Reception 1998–99	Year 2 (2001)
Mild	657	107
Moderate	213	49
Severe	80	7
Profound	37	5
Total	987	168

Box and whisker plots

The data are presented as box and whisker plots. The graph in Figure 6.3 shows three measures of attainment for two groups: the group clustered on the left are scores of children with no hearing loss (none), the group clustered on the right aggregates the scores of all children with a hearing loss. Maths was assessed at the start and end of reception and

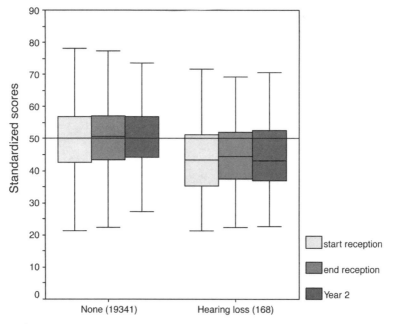

Figure 6.3 Maths and hearing loss. Reception to Year 2 – all pupils.

in Year 2. The horizontal line indicates the mean of 50 for all pupils in PIPS reception and Year 2 assessments – in practice, all non-deaf pupils. Individual pupils can be imagined at points spread along the vertical lines. Half the pupils are spread in each shaded box. The top 25% of pupils are on the line extending from the top of the box to the end. The lowest 25% are on the line extending from the bottom of the rectangle. The shaded rectangle therefore shows the middle 50% of pupils. The median is the black horizontal line inside the box.

Figure 6.3 clearly shows that the aggregated mean scores of pupils with a hearing loss were lower than the group of pupils with no hearing loss on all three measures, although some children with a hearing loss achieved very high scores. It shows that on starting school children with a hearing loss did, on average, attain much lower levels of maths than other children. It shows that by Year 2 levels of attainment were at a similar relative level to those at the start and end of reception.

The graph in Figure 6.4 shows a break down of the aggregated hearing loss group into the four hearing loss categories.

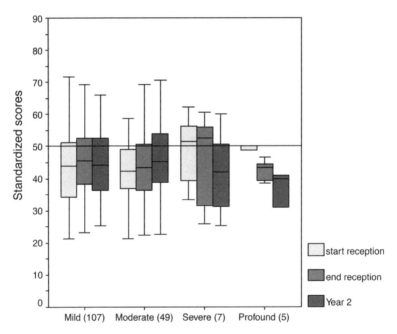

Figure 6.4 Maths and hearing loss. Reception to Year 2.

Maths: mild group

Almost three quarters of this group had scores below 50 at the start of reception, whereas in the normal distribution one would expect half of the group to have scores below 50 and half to have scores above 50. Overall, the scores of this group remained fairly stable between the start of reception and Year 2.

Maths: moderate group

This group showed a similar trend to the mild group.

Maths: severe group

The sample size was very small and it was difficult to make reliable judgements. From the data on the 7 pupils in this category, the maths achievement of children with a severe hearing loss at the start of reception was about average. By Year 2, the median score had dropped to approximately 41.

Maths: profound group

This was the smallest sample of all with just 5 children. At the start of reception, the scores were average but appeared to have dropped by Year 2.

Reading

Measures of reading were analysed for 168 pupils with a hearing loss (Figure 6.5). The middle 50% of aggregated hearing loss pupils progressed as a group relative to the hearing group over the three measurement points. The median at Year 2 was approximately 45.

The graph in Figure 6.5 clearly shows that the aggregated mean scores of pupils with a hearing loss were lower than the group of pupils

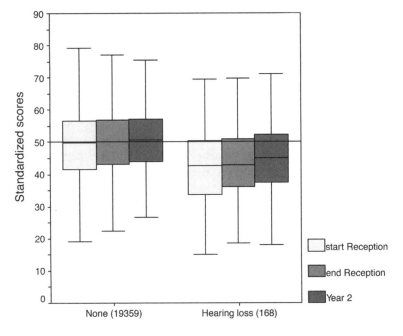

Figure 6.5 Reading and hearing loss. Reception to Year 2 – all pupils.

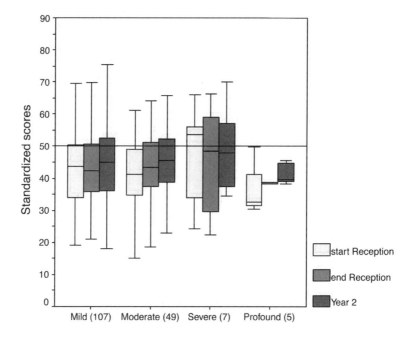

Figure 6.6 Reading and hearing loss. Reception to Year 2.

with no hearing loss on all three measures, although some children with a hearing loss achieved very high scores. It shows that on starting school children with a hearing loss have, on average, attained much lower levels of reading than other children. By Year 2, levels of attainment did, on average, move closer to pupils with no hearing loss. Figure 6.6 shows a breakdown of the aggregated hearing loss group into the four hearing loss categories to look for variation in attainment.

Reading: mild, moderate, severe, profound

The overall trend of the mild group was fairly stable. The moderate group's reading attainment seemed to be increasing – moving closer to the non-hearing loss average – over time. The severe groups' attainment showed signs of becoming stable near the average. The reading of the children in the profound group appeared to be increasing over time from a very low starting point.

Problems of position (POP)

Figure 6.7 shows the same pupils as Figures 6.4 and 6.6. This time it shows their Year 2 POP standardized scores. The means are shown in Table 6.2. The severe group mean was the highest at nearly average, but was for only 7 pupils. The aggregated mean of 46 needs to be considered alongside the POP scores in the next section.

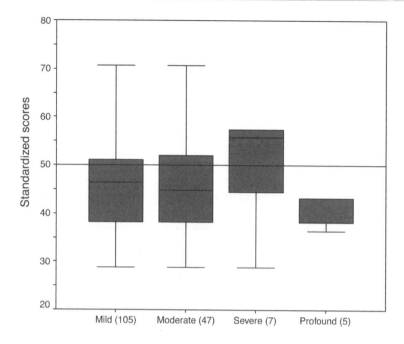

Figure 6.7 POP and hearing loss (Year 2).

Table 6.2 Means of Year 2 POP standardized scores

Hearing loss	Mean score
Mild	46
Moderate	47
Severe	49
Profound	40
Aggregated	46

Teacher effects and culture-reduced assessment

We turn now to the issue of the impact that a teacher can have on a pupil's success on an assessment. Teacher effects due to variation in presentation may be less of an issue for the POP assessment than for language-rich assessment, which involves more teacher input. Even so, teacher effects must surely be present when pupils have not understood what they need to do for the task. The explanation at the beginning must affect pupil's understanding of the task. Once they have understood what is required of them, the culture-reduced characterization of the section is valid, as no further explanation (and therefore language) is involved. Our 'culture-reduced' characterization should have validity across cohorts of pupils using different languages at age-appropriate levels of language development. This should include languages that are signed.

The language attainment per se of pupils may be related to their cognitive development (see MacSweeney, 1998 for a discussion of 'performance' versus 'motor-free' tests and the possible relationship of scores to early knowledge of sign language). Therefore teacher presentation may indeed be connected to the ability to achieve the POP tasks – in the negative sense that understanding by pupils is more difficult for teachers to achieve, even though very little initial explanation is involved.

For January 2001 assessments we had produced our first written and signed guidance for teachers using Year 2 and Year 6 assessments. However, teachers assessed the tracked pupils as described in this section without using our adapted guidance for deaf and hearing-impaired pupils. We rely on teachers contacting the project for guidance to be sent out.

In developing the adapted guidance we had conducted a pilot in April 2000. The numbers using the adapted guidance available generally for Year 2 and Year 6 for the first time in January 2001 were small. The pupils assessed by teachers using the adapted guidance are reported in this section and the following two sections. Before the development of the adapted guidance, information about teacher presentation was not collected. Teachers are now asked to record which presentation they used: spoken English only, BSL, or SSE/sign system.

We felt that it was possible to reliably combine the POP scores of pupils assessed in that 2000 pilot assessment with those who used the guidance in January 2001 as the teachers had used the guidance for this part of the assessment and the teacher presentation was recorded for the first time in both of these. These combined groups at Year 2 and 6 give a larger sample for deaf pupils' averages on this cognitive measure. This larger group also enabled us to look at scores for the first time from the perspective of teacher presentation.

Year 2 and Year 6 POP results

The graphs in Figures 6.8–6.11 show a comparison of Year 2 and Year 6 POP attainments for 91 and 107 pupils respectively, collected with the adapted guidance.

The average POP attainment of the 168 pupils discussed above tracked from reception to Year 2 was approximately 46 (Table 6.2). For the cohorts shown in Figures 6.8–6.11 the mean POP score was just over 49 for Year 2 and just under 49 for Year 6. The lower scores in Figure 6.7 may be due to one or more of the following reasons:

- some pupil's linguistic development may not be age appropriate (in English or BSL or another language)
- some pupil's cognitive ability may be below average
- some pupils may not have understood the initial instructions fully: our guidance was used for the first time with the pupils in the combined groups.

Year 2 mild pupils had the lowest mean POP score (Figure 6.8). The mean scores of the moderate and severe groups were very near to the average for hearing pupils. The profound pupils were exactly average. However, Figure 6.9 shows more variation when the scores are looked at from the perspective of teacher presentation. Teacher presentation by BSL had a median 3 or 4 points above average, with approximately 70% scoring above average. However, there were fewer pupils in this group, which makes the results less reliable.

The bar graph in Figure 6.1 compares hearing loss by teacher presentation for this same group of pupils. We can see that in terms of hearing loss the teachers who used BSL did so with pupils whose hearing loss was either severe or profound. This was also the case with teachers who used SSE/sign system. BSL or SSE/sign system were not used with any pupils in the mild and moderate groups. Of the 57 teachers who used spoken English only, 39 of these were either mild or moderate and 18 were either severe or profound. This provides evidence of a mix of pupil language preferences and school/service policy, but there is also no doubting the effect of severe or profound hearing loss on pupil language preferences (as a reflection of teacher presentation).

The scores of Year 6 pupils can be seen in Figures 6.10 and 6.11. The bar chart in Figure 6.2 shows a very similar distribution of teacher presentation to Year 2. This time the graph of teacher presentation by BSL shows nearly 75% of pupils below average. A two-way analysis of variance test showed a significant interaction between teacher presentation and hearing loss group for the Year 6 POP scores. The severe group achieved significantly higher POP scores when the assessment was presented in BSL and the profound group achieved significantly lower scores when BSL was used compared with SSE. No interaction was found between Year 2 teacher presentation and hearing loss.

Overall the POP sections of Years 2 and 6 show pupils with a hearing loss as generally attaining similarly on this cognitive measure to pupils with no hearing loss. Secondly, when looked at from the perspective of teacher presentation rather than hearing loss, those pupils whose preference (from teacher presentation) was for visual language did not seem to be disadvantaged. Year 2 and 6 POP (measure of cognitive ability) compared by hearing loss and teacher presentation, are shown in Figures 6.8–6.11.

Picture vocabulary for Year 2 and Year 6

This part of the assessment creates a measure of pupil knowledge of English vocabulary. English is either spoken or written. The written word may also be represented in finger-spelling. If teachers use visual gestures to represent any of the English words, then the measure is of something different and is not comparable.

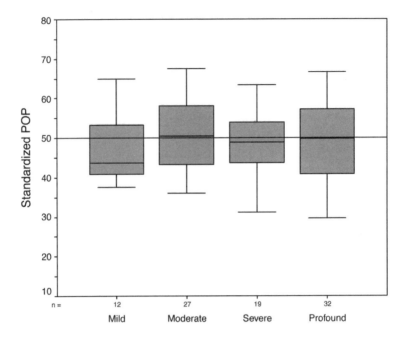

Figure 6.8 POP and hearing loss (Year 2).

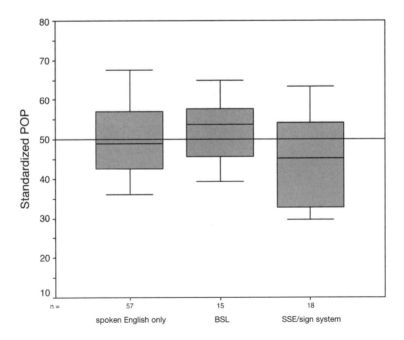

Figure 6.9 POP and teacher presentation (Year 2).

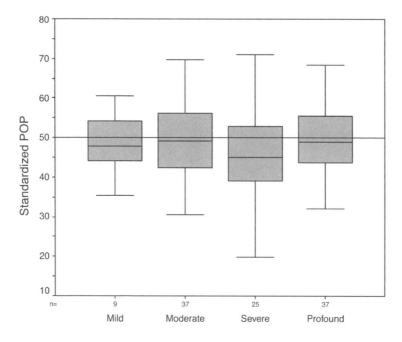

Figure 6.10 POP and hearing loss (Year 6).

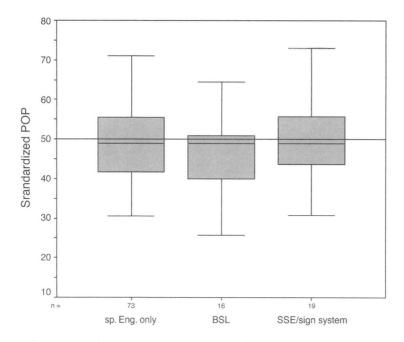

Figure 6.11 POP and teacher presentation (Year 6).

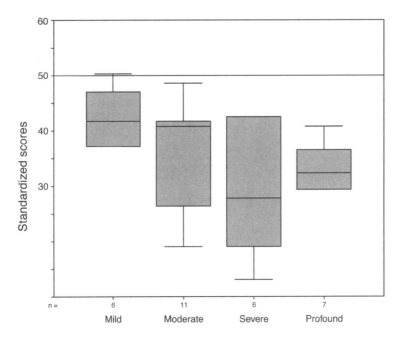

Figure 6.12 Year 2. Picture Vocabulary (English) and hearing loss.

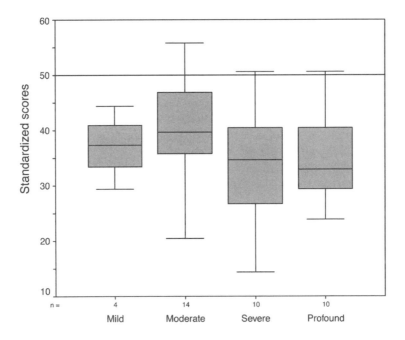

Figure 6.13 Year 6. Picture Vocabulary (English) and hearing loss.

In developing the guidance for deaf and hearing-impaired pupils, some teachers expressed concern that the picture vocabulary would be too difficult for deaf pupils in the severe and profound categories. Some wanted to substitute a sign for the English word and other comments related to the unfairness of this vis-à-vis non-signing pupils. But, as noted above, this would have undermined the purpose of the assessment. Woll has noted:

> [. . .] there are as yet no standardised measures which can be used by professionals working with deaf children to assess their developing competence in sign language. This has resulted in either no assessment of sign language or ad hoc approaches to assessment. (Woll, 1998:65)

(Since then, the 'BSL Language Development: Receptive Skills Test' has been developed; Herman, Holmes and Woll, 1999.) The PIPS assessment explanation and instructions and questions may be given in BSL. The English vocabulary test items are either finger-spelled or pupils are referred to the written words. The assessment of English vocabulary and all the other parts of the assessment can therefore be explained in a way that does not disadvantage pupils who prefer to use a visual language and does not advantage them to other children. The disadvantage for pupils who do prefer to use a visual language is that there is no assessment of this. PIPS do, however, assess knowledge other than English through the medium of BSL.

Figures 6.12 and 6.13 (for Year 2 and 6 respectively) show that deaf pupils in all four categories of hearing loss, on average, achieved lower scores than pupils with no hearing loss. A one-way analysis of variance test showed this difference to be very significant ($p < 0.001$) for both year groups. The numbers were small for each group and therefore need treating with caution. (We could not combine these pupils with the pilot assessments, as the English vocabulary items for the pilot were not identical.) However, for this group the availability of the guidance for teachers gave a degree of confidence that the pupil responses were accurate indications of either reading the printed or finger-spelled word or of listening/lip-reading.

The most common correct raw score was 7 vocabulary items from the 32 for Year 2. For Year 6 it was 12 from 36. For comparison, the most common correct score of pupils with no hearing loss was 18 for Year 2 and 26 for Year 6. The correlation for pupils with a hearing loss is not simply between greater hearing loss and lower attainment. For Year 2 that correlation held until the profound category. For Year 6 the moderate group bucked the trend. Most pupils with a hearing loss did have some knowledge of the vocabulary set, although this was much lower than non-deaf pupils. Nevertheless it was important information that would go unrecorded without the assessment. (It would also render the calculation of value-added inoperable.)

Teacher presentation and subject attainments: Year 2 and Year 6

Figures 6.14 and 6.15 enable us to sketch the outlines of an emerging picture of subject attainments (reading, maths and science) by language use. (Powers, Gregory and Thoutenhoofd, 1998:167) discovered that '. . . there is not a single measure of "linguistic access" in all of the work covered in this review.' The DEMAQS PIPS guidance is a way of ensuring linguistic access at particular points. The data in this and the following sections was gathered by teachers using the guidance to enable them to communicate effectively, in standardized ways, for the assessments. This is a measure at one brief time of linguistic access for these pupils.

Reading and maths were assessed for Year 2. Reading, maths and science were assessed for Year 6. We only have data on 25 pupils for Year 2 and 19 pupils for Year 6. Teacher presentation to 18 pupils in Year 2 and 16 pupils in Year 6 was in spoken English only. Teacher presentation by SSE/sign system was to only 7 and 3 pupils respectively. The subject assessments were optional when registering for PIPS, and this is one of the reasons for the few pupils taking them. Unfortunately, we do not have comparisons where teachers indicated the use of BSL for the presentation. Hopefully we will have these comparisons in future data.

Maths and science assessments are where we might most expect teacher effects; i.e. without teacher guidance and without the signed models of questions for those using BSL or SSE/sign system. For reading, any teacher effect can be expected to be minimal as, after initial instructions, teacher involvement is minimal. However, as with the other subjects, a picture of attainment by teacher presentation/pupil preferred language use is possible.

Pupils could read the questions themselves, or they could be spoken or signed. The pupils of the teachers who indicated they used spoken English only for the administration may have either read the questions themselves, listened or lip-read as the teacher spoke the questions, or both. The teachers who used SSE/sign system were guided with the BSL video models of translated individual questions for vocabulary choice and use of finger-spelling. The results from deaf pupils who used sign language are the first national (i.e. the PIPS cohort in the UK) comparisons for non-deaf and non-signing children on these subjects. They were signing children in that teachers used either BSL or SSE/sign system to present the questions. From Figures 6.1 and 6.2 we know that these pupils were from either the severe or profound groups of pupils.

The graphs show that most of the pupils attained below the national PIPS average on our subject measures. From this small number it seemed attainment was not advantaged or disadvantaged by teacher presentation and, by implication, pupils' preferences for visual language. It needs to be stressed that the statement in the previous sentence is only possible

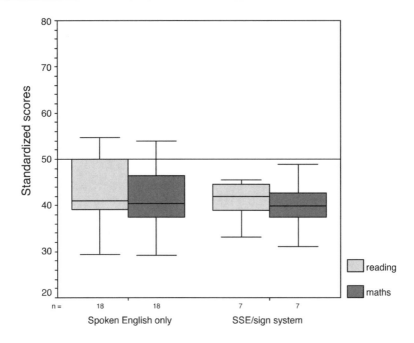

Figure 6.14 Year 2. Teacher presentation and subjects.

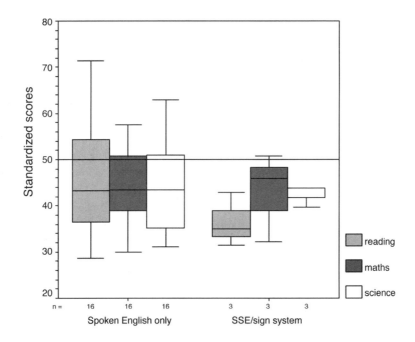

Figure 6.15 Year 6. Teacher presentation and subjects.

because the BSL models of translated questions guided the teachers. We felt that these did standardize the presentation in a similar way to the standardized questions in written English form. We are unable to say more until we have more pupil data on teachers using SSE and BSL. Nevertheless, it is an important principle that educational attainments of pupils are given in terms of language use.

Relative pupil progress: concurrent and prior value-added

The graphs in Figures 6.3–6.6 have enabled us to see the attainments of a cohort of pupils in relation to national norms at three points in time: start and end of reception and Year 2. Figures 6.14–6.18 showed the attainments of pupils in Year 2 and Year 6. However, looking only at attainment gives a somewhat one-dimensional view of pupils. The purpose of the project is to provide teachers with information that is of value to their classroom practice.

The relative progress of individual pupils is calculated by value-added measures. There are two kinds of value-added: prior and concurrent. They differ in what they use to predict a child's present level of attainment. Concurrent value-added uses the child's developed ability to access the National Curriculum (a combination of English vocabulary and cognitive ability) to predict their current level of attainment. It gives us a snapshot of where the child is at this moment in time. By contrast, prior value-added uses the attainment in previous PIPS reading and maths assessments as the predictor. This gives a measure of the child's relative progress over time. To put it another way, concurrent value-added tells us if a child is doing as well, better or worse than expected (given their developed ability) but tells us very little about how they got to that point. Prior value-added tells us something about the child's progress since the last PIPS assessment but little about whether we can expect them to do better still. The calculation and interpretation of concurrent and prior value-added scores is explained in more detail in Tymms and Albone, 2002: see also the PIPS website (*http://www.cem.dur.ac.uk/pips*).

The DEMAQS PIPS guidance is a way of ensuring linguistic access at particular points. The data in this section and the previous one was gathered by teachers using the guidance to enable them to communicate effectively, in standardized ways, for the assessments. This is a measure at one brief time of linguistic access for these pupils.

Using value-added: five pupil examples

Tables 6.3 and 6.4 show attainments placed in a context of pupil progress as predicted by cognitive ability and picture vocabulary (concurrent value-added) and previous assessment (prior value-added). The concurrent and prior rows each show a value-added calculation (the residual) – the closer the number to zero, the closer the pupil attainment to what was predicted. Plus or minus 5 are the upper and lower limits of expected value-added. The last but one column shows teacher presentation to highlight language use. The final column shows hearing loss as an important individual characteristic with a learning implication.

Five examples from those same Year 2 and Year 6 pupils are given in Table 6.3. For each pupil a subject score is given along with (English) picture vocabulary and POP scores. The latter, picture vocabulary and POP, form the basis of the construct 'developed ability' from which a concurrent value-added score is calculated. As the adapted guidance was used for the Year 2 and Year 6 assessments we are confident about the reliability of the calculation of concurrent value-added. However, the prior value-added calculation needs treating with caution, as no guidance was available for the previous assessment.

Table 6.3 Attainments placed in a context of pupil progress: two Year 6 pupils

Pupil		Maths	Reading	Science	Picture	POP vocabulary	Teacher presentation	Hearing loss
6A	Attainment	45.80	38.08	50.27	40.40	41.65	Spoken English	Severe
	Concurrent	2.33	−5.17	7.16				
	Prior	5.55	−1.71	9.50				
6B	Attainment	45.80	35.03	43.88	31.88	49.13	SSE/sign system	Profound
	Concurrent	5.80	−4.66	4.41				
	Prior	.97	−9.52	−1.13				

Pupil 6A

This pupil was almost one standard deviation below the average (50) on POP and similarly with picture vocabulary. For the subjects, science was average and maths was 4 points below average. Reading attainment was low at 38. The second row shows the concurrent value-added and the last row prior value-added. The pupil's maths attainment of almost 46 when measured against developed ability gave a positive residual of 2.33. Therefore this pupil was performing more or less as predicted in maths. The pupil's reading was below expected attainment, but science was above. The pupil's teachers would be able to integrate these findings with their own much more intimate knowledge of the pupil. The value-added assessments are a tool to support the professional judgement of teachers.

This pupil also had value-added from a prior PIPS assessment. The combination of prior and concurrent value-added can provide a richer view of pupil progress. This pupil has an interesting pattern of subject progress. Maths prior was also positive and therefore consistent with concurrent. Science concurrent and prior possibly indicates some previous underachievement followed by good progress. Low attainment in reading alongside slightly negative prior value-added and a higher negative concurrent indicates English was difficult for this pupil. Teachers may use this evidence to review pupil support.

Pupil 6B

This pupil had an average POP score. We can see this may accompany a very low picture vocabulary and low reading scores (both English attainments) but maths and science knowledge may be relatively much higher. Prior value-added for maths and science show progress almost as predicted. Concurrent shows better than predicted performance. This indicates good progress and movement closer to national norms on these two attainments.

The low reading attainment (35) and value-added (concurrent −4.66, prior −9.52) indicated that the pupil is underachieving and falling further behind. Teacher presentation was SSE/sign system and the pupil's hearing loss category was profound. This is where the debate over BSL comes to the fore. Teacher presentation combined with the low reading attainment indicated that the pupil more readily understands a signed language.

Table 6.4 Attainments placed in a context of pupil progress: three Year 2 pupils

Pupil		Maths	Reading	Picture	POP vocabulary	Teacher presentation	Hearing loss
2A	Attainment	39.86	45.53	40.83	43.23	SSE / sign system	Profound
	Concurrent	−4.42	0.84				
	Prior	−5.16	0.76				
2B	Attainment	32.50	39.52	23.38	57.36	Spoken English	Moderate
	Concurrent	−9.24	−2.81				
	Prior	−	−				
2C	Attainment	37.53	29.36	37.14	49.57	Spoken English	Mild
	Concurrent	−6.76	−15.34				
	Prior	−0.15	−7.76				

Pupil 2A

This pupil, from Year 2, had a maths score of 40 with negative concurrent and prior value-added. Both measures showed that attainment in maths was below expected, indicating continuing underachievement. Reading attainment was slightly below average, with value-added indicating the pupil was achieving as expected for both assessments. The pupil's teachers would need to confirm this.

Pupil 2A had a hearing loss diagnosed at 6–12 months and a cochlear implant at age 3. Class support is regularly a *'signing non-teaching assistant'* and 2 hours weekly with a Teacher of the Deaf (ToD). The teacher commented that, *'Initially signing was used for all "verbal" communication but as the child's hearing and vocabulary develops signing is being used as a back up'*. However, the teacher also wrote about the assessment: *'Because it was something new [the pupil] relied heavily on signing for the test rather than listening and used signing as a back up'*. This indicated that the pupil's educational knowledge was still being acquired with signing. Rather than being accepted as the pupil's preferred language – for ease of acquiring knowledge and communication – signing was viewed as a prop that would eventually not be needed. The value-added data, along with other factors, provide valuable information for the school regarding the educational approach for this pupil.

Pupil 2B

This pupil was not involved in previous PIPS and therefore does not have prior value-added. The pupil was above average for cognitive ability but the picture vocabulary score was very low. Reading attainment was also low at 40. Maths attainment was exceptionally low. Concurrent value-added indicates this pupil was underachieving in maths. Reading value-added was almost at the predicted level.

The evidence of this assessment would be important input to the pupil's SEN (Special Educational Needs) process and IEP (Individual Education Plan). At the time of the assessment the pupil was at Stage 3. This pupil was in the regular class for 100% of the timetable, following the same curriculum with no disapplied, modified or additional subjects. A support assistant was allocated to work with the pupil 'individually and in small groups' for 50% of the time. From teacher presentation, it seemed the pupil was monolingual in English.

This pupil was diagnosed as having a moderate hearing loss at the late age of between age 5 and 6. This pupil's assessment will be of concern to the school. The pupil had a better than average cognitive ability. The low English attainment, as also evidenced with the picture vocabulary, was very likely related to the pupil not being picked up as having a hearing loss. Because maths ability is entwined with language development, the low vocabulary and reading scores possibly impacted on maths.

Pupil 2C

This pupil was identified as having a mild hearing loss at 5–6 years of age, was at stage 3 for SEN and was visited by a peripatetic ToD for

30–60 minutes per week. The pupil's POP score was average, reading very low at 30 and maths low at 38. Reading value-added gives rise to concern. Prior (–8) and concurrent (–15) indicates a greater falling off in what was very low attainment. Progress in maths is also well below prediction by concurrent value-added. Overall, considering both concurrent and prior value-added, there had been a marked deterioration in this pupil's progress.

Summary and conclusions

Guidance was developed to standardize the administration of assessments to pupils with hearing loss. Guidance was both written and in BSL. Teachers using spoken English only for assessments with deaf pupils seemed to do so always with pupils with mild or moderate hearing loss. The written guidance and BSL translations now enable attainments to be administered appropriately for individual pupils. This controls for when (or when not) to use finger-spelled words and for BSL sign vocabulary choices. This was also crucial for teachers who indicated they used SSE/sign system for presentation. The results from deaf pupils who use sign language are the first UK comparisons we have with non-deaf and non-signing children on these subjects. They are signing children in that teachers used either BSL or SSE/sign system to present the questions.

Two sets of pupil data, at Year 2 and Year 6, were compared on a cognitive assessment to national norms. The Year 2 POP scores of the tracked cohort differed by almost one third of a SD from the Year 2 scores of pupils whose teachers used guidance specifically designed for assessing deaf and hearing-impaired pupils. These same pupils' cognitive ability scores were also investigated along an additional dimension – that of teacher presentation. Year 2 and Year 6 subject attainments were also looked at by teacher presentation. This was found to be a useful additional perspective from which to view pupil attainment and progress – as a reflection of pupil language preferences and regular teaching approach.

Examples of Year 2 and Year 6 pupil attainments were placed in the context of concurrent and prior value-added in reading, maths and science (the latter at Year 6 only). Maths and science are the areas where teacher presentation is more significant for pupil responses as they contain individual questions with high cultural effects. POP and (English) picture vocabulary both have a large number of individual assessment items, but the teacher effect is confined to being at the initial stage of explanation or instruction. The subject assessments of maths and science are different. If the teacher is presenting each question (rather than the pupil only reading it) then teacher effects may be high if guidance is not adhered to.

When the graphs in Figures 6.14 and 6.15 (Reading, Year 2 and Year 6) are compared, viewed from the perspective of teacher presentation, it is evident that there is a gap between pupils with a hearing loss and the PIPS national average. However, these were two different cohorts of pupils and they are our first comparisons between spoken English only and signing pupils. Little more can be said until we gather more data and track more pupils through their primary years. Figures 6.16 and 6.17 (maths, Year 2 and Year 6) and Figure 6.18 (science, Year 6) show a similar gap between our pupils and the PIPS national average. However, for pupils with a hearing loss, between Year 2 and Year 6, attainment levels on average do not seem to become closer to the national average. This was also the case for the cohort tracked from reception to Year 2. For reading, however, there was some rise in attainment (Figure 6.5).

The prediction of concurrent value-added was based on developed ability. Attainment in a prior assessment was used as an additional value-added measure. The individual pupil examples gave us a mixed evaluation of the findings. Further evidence is needed before we can say whether the average value-added of deaf and hearing-impaired pupils is constant or shows that these pupils fall further behind over time.

There is one important ability variable missing for some of these pupils – their communicative competence. Knowledge of sign language is not being assessed yet it had to be taken into account for the creation of reliable assessments. Some of the pupils clearly have knowledge of sign language and their teachers feel they must use this to communicate with these pupils. Their curriculum knowledge is therefore acquired by signing. The only way PIPS could reliably assess these pupils was to produce standardized instructions and questions for teachers. This pupil ability is consistently ignored for most official education purposes. The approach used at the moment for administering SATs (the Standard Attainment Tasks used to test the progress of English schoolchildren at intervals during the school years) is unreliable. Written guidance is produced but schools and teachers are left to translate it into signed language. The Qualifications and Curriculum Authority produce 'Special arrangements for the tests' (see the QCA website, *http://www.qca.org.uk/ca/tests/ara/ks2_special.asp*).

The only way to produce reliable, standardized assessments in signed language is for those assessments to be produced independently. Unlike the use of a first spoken language, the use of sign language as a first/preferred language does not decrease with age. There will be a continuing need for standardized assessments in sign language.

National standardized assessments of pupils classified by hearing loss are now possible from a perspective of language use – defined by teacher presentation. The pupil's particular hearing loss is seen as an individual characteristic reported alongside other characteristics that may affect pupil attainments and progress. The monolingual (either

English or BSL) or bilingual (English and BSL) abilities and preferences of pupils are then highlighted for teachers, schools and parents. This perspective does not downgrade the 'deaf or Deaf' identity aspect of children, but it does highlight language use in an educational context.

The overall reasons that attainments were below national standards are linked by language and hearing loss. As suggested above, there are specific ways to improve schools and service support related to individual pupils. On average, pupils with a hearing loss enter school with lower early reading and early maths attainments than other pupils. It seems reasonable to conclude that one way to improve overall average attainments of pupils with hearing loss on entering compulsory schooling is to identify those children before compulsory education and then to provide parents and child with ongoing adequate and appropriate educational support in the home. Parents generally have positive attitudes toward universal neonatal hearing screening (UNHS). Of four key reasons identified, one is, 'parents whose children are identified as deaf report welcoming the opportunity for intervention to start as early as possible'. (Young and Andrews, 2001:153) As identified in this research, the support needs to be around general aspects of child learning and particular aspects of language (BSL and/or English) acquisition for the early development of literacy and maths.

Acknowledgements

David Brien of the former Deaf Studies Research Unit, University of Durham was responsible with Peter Tymms for the original development of the DEMAQS Project. Judith Collins, Department of Linguistics and English Language, University of Durham is consultant for BSL and responsible for translations of assessments. The PIPS team at the Curriculum, Evaluation and Management Centre, University of Durham are responsible for the initial value-added data analysis of the pupils in this chapter.

Chapter 7
Sign bilingual deaf children's writing strategies: responses to different sources for writing

RUTH SWANWICK

Proponents of sign bilingual education for deaf children propose that deaf children's developing skills in BSL will provide a foundation for their subsequent English language development, including literacy skills (Rodda and Eleweke, 2000). Sign bilingual deaf children should therefore approach the learning of literacy with sign language skills through which English language learning can be mediated. In practical terms we still need to know more about how to use both languages in the teaching context and how to bridge the gap between the two languages (Albertini, 2000; Musselman, 2000). How best to use sign language and (spoken or written) English for the teaching of English to deaf children is a question frequently posed by teachers. Pupils need access to and experience of English, but also explanation and discussion in sign language. These learning and teaching issues provide the focus for this chapter.

The term 'sign bilingual' is used here to describe deaf children and adults who are bilingual in a spoken and a signed language such as English and BSL (Pickersgill and Gregory, 1998). The current use of this term in the educational context allows deaf pupils' educational needs to be considered within a broad bilingual framework but for their specific learning needs related to their cross-modal bilingualism to be recognized, including access to both languages, code mixing and transfer from one modality to another.

This chapter looks at one area of data from a larger study into deaf children's developing sign bilingualism. This aspect of the study focused specifically on ways in which deaf children apply their knowledge and experience of British Sign Language (BSL) to the task of writing in English. Samples of young deaf children's writing in response

121

to a BSL story and a picture sequence were compared and an analysis was made of the role of BSL in the writing process. Similarities between the children's written responses to these two sources were identified, notably the increased complexity of their written grammatical structures used in the translation task and the problems encountered in moving between the sign and written modalities. Different ways in which individuals applied their knowledge of BSL to the writing task and deployed their English resources were also identified, leading to a discussion of the implications for the teaching of literacy to bilingual deaf children.

Deaf children's attainments in writing

Deaf children's performance in literacy is very well documented, but the majority of reports reference deaf children's achievements to hearing models of literacy development and pedagogy. This body of research provides a useful framework for considering literacy development but it is not comprehensive, since many deaf children use sign language and are learning English as a second or additional language. Although many of the findings regarding deaf children's difficulties may be relevant to all deaf children (Paul, 1998), investigations into literacy from this cultural and linguistic perspective are more likely to reveal the different learning styles and strategies of sign bilingual deaf children.

Deaf children's attainments in the domain of writing reflect the difficulties they experience with the reading process (Powers, Gregory and Thoutenhoofd, 1998; Wilbur, 2000). The focus of research attention has been largely on errors in deaf children's writing, and these have been catalogued extensively. The most significant areas of difficulty reported for deaf children are limited written vocabulary and insecure grasp of written English syntax. Typical errors reported are incorrect use of word order, omission of function words and omission or incorrect use of inflectional morphology such as plurality, verb agreement or tense (Lichtenstein, 1998). Explanations for these problems have focused largely on deaf children's early linguistic experiences and access to spoken English, but some researchers have also raised questions about teaching approaches and the extent to which they contribute to deaf children's writing problems. High levels of teacher management and control that focus on the structure of written English, rather than on pupils' abilities to reflect and discuss, have been identified as constraining the literacy development of deaf pupils rather than guiding and facilitating it (Lane, Hoffmeister and Bahan, 1996; Paul, 1998; Webster and Heineman-Gosschalk, 2000). Wilbur (2000) for example, identifies teacher focus on sentence structure as a possible explanation for deaf children's stilted writing style which 'lacks complexity and creativity in terms of temporal sequence' (2000:83).

Deaf children writing in a second language

It is a concern that, as with research into the reading process, the majority of research into deaf children's writing fails to identify their different linguistic skills and capabilities. It has been established that deaf children's writing is not a reflection of their manual communication skills (Everhart and Marschark, 1988), nor is it an indication of their general cognitive abilities (Yoshinaga-Itano and Snyder, 1985). Everhart and Marschark point out that these findings suggest that deaf children are capable of achieving literacy success, and this is good cause to question the research and teaching approaches.

A small number of studies have considered deaf children's writing from a different perspective in that they have sought to identify what is different about their writing abilities and whether these differences are specific to deaf children (Charrow and Fletcher, 1974; Goldberg and Bordman, 1975; Baker, 1994; Gregory, 1997). This perspective considers that deaf children's errors may be explained by the influence of sign language on their writing, and hence provide evidence of an attempt to create their own structures using a language that they already know.

Some researchers have looked specifically for evidence of the influence of sign language on bilingual deaf children's literacy development. An early study by Jones (1979) of deaf students' texts showed that these students were not translating non-manual signs when writing (e.g. use of facial expression, body movement) but tended instead to provide a gloss of the manual signs. Jones suggests that this points to a lack of awareness of the importance of the non-manual signals. Because of this, the original sign language message was not sufficiently conveyed through the students' text to allow it to be comprehensible.

Jones argues that this problem may arise because the students consider that sign language, like English, has one primary channel through which all information is encoded. These findings focus on what is missed out of the written form but give no information about ways in which deaf children are constructing their model of written English other than to suggest that they attempt to write down a manual gloss of Pidgin Sign English.

In contrast to this, more recent research suggests that errors in deaf children's writing illustrate their attempts to creatively invent language structures using the blueprint of a language that they already know (Gregory, 1997). Gregory's study is one of the few that considers deaf children's writing strategies and achievements from a second language perspective where BSL is recognized as the preferred language and it is acknowledged that written English is likely to be the main means of access to English. This research considered the strategies the children used for writing and the extent to which their knowledge of BSL influenced their writing, in both positive (facilitative) and negative (interference) terms. Gregory concludes from the analysis of the children's errors that deaf children use their knowledge of BSL in their English writing. Gregory argues that this should be considered as a positive transitional stage, which could open up the possibilities of the use of BSL for the discussion of English and how it expresses grammatical information in comparison to sign language.

Mayer and Wells (1996) discuss bilingual deaf children's literacy development from a theoretical viewpoint. They outline the mental processes involved in preparing thoughts and ideas in sign language and writing them down in English. The central problem they raise concerning deaf children's experience of writing is that of the interdependence between the spoken and written forms of English, namely the role of inner speech. Inner speech is seen as an intermediary between oral speech and writing. This is not to say that text is speech written down, but that inner speech is a means to rehearse, self-direct and mediate the writing process. Inner speech is associated with oral speech and this leads us to ask whether all deaf children will have this facility. However, there is evidence to suggest that some deaf children do have inner language based on the visual-gestural properties of sign language.

Mayer and Wells (1996) suggest that because of this difference in modality deaf children might experience particular difficulties in moving from a mental representation in sign language to the written form.

They illustrate this point by identifying the types of problems that deaf children are likely to experience when translating between a sign language and a written language where they encounter information in one language that is not specified the same way in the other language. For example, adverbial information is often conveyed in BSL through the way in which a sign is produced, whereas in English an adverb can be specified using an actual word.

In asking deaf learners to translate from BSL to written English it may be that the process is further complicated. In doing this, we are imposing a source language of sign language which may inhibit their abilities to retrieve whatever inner representation of the spoken language they might have. Since much of deaf children's writing experience in bilingual settings does involves some preparatory work in BSL, the advantages and disadvantages of this common practice need to be further explored.

Relationship between first- and second-language writing

This question over the extent to which the learner's first language influences their second-language writing strategies also extends to hearing learners of English as a second or additional language (L2). Research into second-language writing concludes that children learn to read and write only once, and that there is therefore a strong relationship between the process of writing in a native language (L1) and writing in a second language (Krapels, 1990). The basic principle proposed is that L1 writing ability provides second-language learners with linguistic resources to use as they approach L2 writing (Hudelson, 1989). This relationship, sometimes viewed as 'interference', can be more usefully constructed as 'application'. This different perspective emphasizes that L2 writers can usefully apply their tacit knowledge of writing in the L1 to writing in the L2 (Edelsky, 1982).

This transfer of strategies has been found to occur even where the two languages are kept separate in an attempt to avoid interference; it is therefore not a phenomenon restricted to translation activities (Friedlander, 1990). Indeed, Uzawa (1996) suggests that second-language writing and translation tasks involve the same cognitive processes. Language learners have been found to use their first language or translation as a stage in the process of writing in their second language as a means of compensating for their lack of vocabulary. Other positive effects of L1 transfer include the use of L1 for generating topic information (Cumming, 1987), and the use of code switching to increase options for meaning-making (Edelsky and Jilbert, 1985).

In considering bilingual deaf children's experience of writing, we cannot look to their primary experience of writing. They will approach the writing of English without prior experience of learning to write in their primary language, and with limited access the spoken form of the language they are writing down. Although they may have developed sign language as a primary language and have age-appropriate conversational skills, developing literacy proficiency involves learning processes that are qualitatively different from those involved in primary language development (Francis, 1999). Literacy learning involves higher-order processes associated with a reflection on language structures that are essentially distinct from the primary and universal development of first language competence. Whereas face-to-face interaction (oral discourse) allows for active negotiation, writing is essentially non-reciprocal activity which depends less on the extralinguistic situation and more on the reflective and deliberate use of text as the source of information (Olson, 1996).

Research questions

This body of research into bilingualism and literacy raises an interesting question for deaf learners. Given that they do not have prior writing skills to apply to English writing, to what extent do they apply their linguistic resources (spoken and signed) to the writing process? This chapter considers what can be learnt about sign bilingual children's experience of the writing process through an analysis of their strategies for writing English stories in response to a BSL source (translation writing) and a picture source (non-translation writing).

Subjects

Six 7- and 8-year old children, in two bilingual settings (three children in each) were selected as subjects for the study because they all used both BSL and English for learning and for socializing at home and at school, and so could be considered to be bilingual to varying degrees. These children were also all in a bilingual educational programme where deaf and hearing adults worked together and where both BSL and English (spoken and written) were used in the teaching situation. The children had varying degrees of hearing loss and although this is considered in the analysis, the main criterion for the choice of the subjects was the functional use of both languages in the learning context.

Research context

The research took place within an inclusive education support service for deaf pupils, which has a sign bilingual policy. This support service promotes the role of deaf adults and BSL in the education of deaf children. The development and use of BSL is encouraged through the employment of deaf native users and hearing staff proficient in sign language.

Research approach rationale

The exploratory nature of this study embraces a grounded approach to the development of our understanding of the little-understood phenomenon of sign bilingualism. The most relevant theoretical basis for this work is the body of research into the language skills of bilingual hearing children. However, because of the differences that sign bilingualism entails it is not appropriate simply to seek to verify any one of these theories, although this established conceptual framework was used to develop an appropriate methodology. The conclusions drawn from this study are therefore grounded in that they arise from the interpretation of the data (Glaser and Strauss, 1967).

A set of six individual exploratory case studies with clearly defined techniques for data collection was used in this investigation. We recognize that studying six case studies rather than one will not lead to opportunities to generalize about all sign bilingual children but that different results will be achieved which will facilitate the generation of a theory about their language learning strategies (Robson, 1993; Yin, 1989).

Although the researcher worked with the individual children on the data collection activities, the teachers of the children played a significant role in planning and reviewing these. The teachers were interested in learning more about the children's linguistic potential so that they might adapt and develop their teaching strategies. The collaborative nature of this study points to an action research approach as the project aims to address some of the practical concerns of teachers regarding the teaching of English (Stenhouse, 1985).

Pilot project

The exploratory pilot work prompted the development of some pre-structured data collection techniques. The pilots provided a preliminary guide as to what might be expected to emerge from the data collection and what the researcher should be looking for. The pilot work yielded information about the individual deaf children's language learning strategies and language awareness. The analysis of this provided indications of what sort of structured language activities would stretch this potential in each child and provide further evidence of these strategies (Swanwick, 2001).

One of the far-reaching findings from the pilot studies concerned the individual nature of each deaf child's bilingualism and the impossibility of evolving clearly defined categories which might be generalizable to all sign bilingual children. This factor prescribed the need for richly descriptive case studies to be developed to discuss each individual's bilingualism with the intention of identifying issues that would be significant for all sign bilingual children. A need for qualitative data was therefore identified, as this type of data is more likely to provide insight into behaviours and processes than quantitative data. The qualitative data collected is intended to provide a snapshot of individual children's experiences of learning and moving between two languages which will inform continued research and development in sign bilingual education.

Elicitation techniques

This aspect of the study involved the use of two linguistic manipulation tasks of translation and non-translation writing. The language demands of each activity reflected the typical language demands placed on the children in the school setting, although the activities necessarily concentrated this experience for the purposes of the research. The structured tasks were intended to elicit richer and more concentrated data about the processes of language learning than unstructured observation would yield.

Writing from a BSL story source

The children were asked to view a BSL story on video being told by a familiar native sign language user. This was done on a 1:1 basis with the researcher. The children were asked to watch the story and write their English version. The tape was reviewed as often as they requested. Any help they requested was given and noted.

Writing from a picture story source

To provide a contrast and a control for the written outcomes of the translation activity, the children were also asked to write a story from a short sequence of pictures. This activity was intended to provide an opportunity to contrast the children's writing from two different sources so that BSL influences on the children's writing might be identified. This work had been previously piloted with the children by their teachers in the two groups, which informed decisions about the appropriate length of the BSL and the written story.

This activity took place 2 months after the translation activity. The assumption made was that this was a 'language free' source and that this would result in differences between the children's two written stories. Whether or not this assumption was a valid one is considered after the analysis of the individual results. Certainly it can be argued that the picture story source might allow the children to make their own interpretations and language choices to a greater extent than the BSL story. It might therefore be assumed that the picture source would result in more confident and complex writing from the children as they can choose to use the best of their English repertoire.

Instructions were given to the individual pupils in their preferred mode of communication. At the beginning of each activity the children were asked if they preferred the researcher to use voice and sign, voice only or sign only.

Focus of analysis

Because this was part of a wider study of sign bilingualism, of an exploratory and grounded nature, a formal linguistic analysis procedure was not used although areas for analysis were identified. We anticipated that this aspect of analysis would indicate in the first instance whether or not any significant differences were evident between the children's different texts. We anticipated that these findings would then facilitate the development of an appropriate analysis tool.

We considered that the two tasks would require the children to approach writing from two different starting points and that the results would therefore lead to some useful preliminary conclusions. We compared the two texts to examine to what extent the children's translation text was influenced by the BSL source, where they benefited from the BSL source as compared to a picture-sequence source and where they may have been disadvantaged. The areas considered included

- difference in word length
- difference in types of grammatical structures
- range of vocabulary used.

It was not possible to match the two stimuli exactly because of the different modes in which they were presented (BSL and pictures), but a match was made in terms of story genre, structure and length. The children were allowed to ask for help with the vocabulary in both writing activities, since asking them to do unsupported writing was not a normal classroom procedure. The help that the children requested was therefore considered in the analysis in relation to their final written outcome.

For the purposes of the analysis and discussion, two children's contrasting texts are presented in Figures 7.1–7.4, exactly as written by the children including line breaks, spelling, punctuation and use of capitals and lower-case letters. Beneath the two contrasting texts for each child, a brief summary of the individual analysis is given before specific findings relating to all of the children's text are discussed. The examples described below illustrate the contrasting approaches to this writing task which were observed across the full group of six children.

'Josh and BiLLy'
Josh got a new dog its NaMe BiLLy.
Josh got a idea for DADDY BirtHday Cake.
BiLLy was HaPPy to buy the Cake.
Josh was waiting for DADDy back
DADDy was back Josh said COME here
there you are it disappear DADDy saw BiLLy
got a chocolate round Billy mouh.

Figure 7.1 Hannah. Text written from BSL story.

'The big box'
Chip and Biff Look at the box.
Biff got a idea. Biff Paint the box.
and mum cut the box.
Chip was Happy Kipper can't see.
Floppy was Happy too. then mum
came then mum was shocked
about the box. Kipper was Happy
Biff was Happy Chip was Happy
again.

Figure 7.2 Hannah. Text written from picture sequence.

Both of Hannah's texts were approximately the same length but there was a marked difference between the grammatical structures she used in her BSL translation text and her picture-based text. The structures used in the translation text were much more complex than those in the picture-based text, characterized by her use of subordinate clauses. This attempt to write more complex English in response to the translation activity was common to all six children. Although there were twice as many errors in Hannah's translation text, overall it also introduced many more new ideas and avoided repetition. The comparison text involved more repetitive structures. This repetitive style was also a feature of the other children's picture-based writing. The BSL source seems to have influenced Hannah's use of structures and vocabulary because she appeared to be highly motivated to express the equivalent meanings in her writing even though at times they exceeded her English grammatical knowledge. This suggests that her errors were not a result of her trying to write down a gloss of the BSL, but perhaps errors made in an attempt to use unfamiliar and complex written English structures.

> Hi My little son billy new.
> dog want come with in shoP.
> better leave house went to shoP look
> around idea make chocolate cake.
> Chocolate cake leave smell nice
> wait for DaDDy at last home
> cake gone where dog chocolate
> all over his mouth

Figure 7.3 Lucy. Text written from BSL story.

> biff and Chip Put up the a
> box mummy Help too
> biff Paint the a roof
> mummy cuts the door
> biff and chip and Kipper in
> the house
> the house is melting
> because is raining
> now is got a new
> tent

Figure 7.4 Lucy. Text written from picture sequence.

Both of Lucy's texts were approximately the same length. The use of English grammar conventions and the style of Lucy's translation text seem to be markedly influenced by the BSL version of the story. This text is a written gloss of the BSL in so far as this is possible. Interestingly, this approach to writing was adopted by all the children in the group with less well-developed spoken English abilities. The text lacks written English structure because of this but, nonetheless, all of the key ideas in the story are there. This suggests that the BSL version of the story did interfere in some way with Lucy's ability to draw on the English grammatical knowledge that she demonstrates in the picture-based text. Lucy had perhaps not re-thought the BSL story in English before attempting to write it down. Being able to do this seemed to be related to the children's ability to use spoken English to plan their writing. This effect on Lucy could indicate that BSL is her stronger language, as she was unable to impose her knowledge of English on the BSL source.

General features of the children's writing

All of the children's texts were considered in this way. From this initial analysis it was found that some writing strategies, characteristics and problems were common to all, or most, of the children despite their diverse linguistic abilities.

The most notable trend was that the children generally used more complex grammatical structures in their translation texts than in their picture-source texts. Characteristically the complex structures found in the translation texts included:

- the use of subordinate clauses such as *Billy was happy to buy the cake*
- complex noun phrases such as *daddy birthday cake*
- connective clauses such as *look around idea make chocolate cake*

By contrast, the structures used in the picture-based texts were more usually short, simple main clauses such as *Chip was happy* or simple clauses without a subject as in *paint the box* and these were often conjoined by *and* or *then*

Another similarity with regard to the children's writing style was the amount of repetition found in the picture-source texts. When the children had to draw on their own English resources to write the picture-based text they seemed to rely more heavily on the repetitive use of the characters' names and on the frequent use of *then* to conjoin clauses. In the translation text they generally did not repeat themselves in this way. The BSL story source perhaps pushed them beyond their learnt writing strategies and focus on sentence structure, as identified by Wilbur (2000), and challenged their creative use of written English.

A further interesting challenge for all of the children was how to address the different styles of a written English and a live BSL story and how to convey this in their writing. The children clearly already had strategies for writing an English story from the narrator's perspective. They were aware that they had to identify characters and describe events in a logical sequence and indicate who is doing what. However, the BSL story as the source presented particular problems for their writing because of the discrepancies between the visual and written modalities. In the BSL version the storyteller represented the characters and the subject was rarely named but indicated through role shift and placement. Some of the children tried to write in the style in which the BSL story was told, in that they told the story as the participant. This is most marked at the start of the story where the deaf narrator sets the scene and the children attempted to recreate this in their writing as in *Hi My little son billy new dog*. This influence on their writing style continued, with the result that the subject was often omitted or only a single subject was specified for connective clauses in the translation texts as in *chocolate leave smell nice*. Also, names, subject pronouns, definite and indefinite articles were often omitted in the translation texts even though the children demonstrated an understanding of their usage in their picture-based texts.

Individual writing strategies

These general features raise several issues about the role of BSL in the teaching of English and the respective value of these contrasting writing activities in a bilingual literacy programme. A closer look at individual approaches broadens this discussion since it became apparent from the analysis of all the texts that each child brings a diverse repertoire of bilingual abilities to the writing task. There was no one process that could be applied to all of the children and yet there are some indications of why certain individuals might have deployed their bilingual skills in particular ways.

Role of spoken English in the writing process

The children, such as Hannah, who demonstrated some ability to mentally prepare their writing using their spoken language skills, seemed to be able to retain their sense of English in the translation situation. These children's texts did not differ significantly. For these children English was probably their stronger language. The way in which they were affected by the BSL source was more a matter of motivation to convey the sense of the story and a reflection of the fact that they had not set their own language boundaries, as they can do in the picture-based text. It should also be noted that the BSL source forced the children to ask for more help that may have resulted in a more complex written product from some.

Role of BSL in the writing process

From this initial analysis it seems that the children with less well-developed spoken language skills, such as Lucy, tended to write down a gloss of the BSL in response to the translation writing activity. The difference between their two texts are therefore more marked because of the stronger influence of the BSL in the translation text, which is less evident in the picture-based text. This leads us to interesting and useful information about different bilingual deaf children's starting points for writing in English.

The findings so far lead us to speculate that the translation task was a different activity for each individual, depending on their starting point. For the deaf children without strong spoken language skills the actual writing was more like the first stage of the translation process. The writing of the gloss of the BSL provided a link from the BSL to the written English, thus allowing them to commence the writing and then incorporate their own English knowledge as appropriate. This supports findings from other studies, which stress the value of using a written gloss as an intermediary between ASL or BSL and written English (Mozzer-Mather, 1990; Neuroth-Gimbrone and Logiodice, 1992; Singleton et al, 1998).

For the children with more spoken English skills, the writing down of the English was more like the end of the translation process. It seems that translation for these children took place internally, enabling them to then verbalize their English version before writing. It is likely that the children with more developed spoken language skills had a model of written English that is more similar to that of hearing children. Consequently, these children seemed to be thinking and planning in English in preparation for writing. As a result, their written texts successfully conveyed the sense of the BSL story but were not hidebound by the structure of the BSL source. Their internal model of English thus enabled them to be more proficient writers, confirming other similar reports (Mayer, 1999; Mayer and Akamatsu, 2000).

Influence of the source on the writing process

Five out of the six children all produced more examples of correct English in their picture-based texts. It seems to be a combination of factors that created this contrast between these children's texts.

First of all, they were perhaps driven to try to express the complexities of the BSL story in whatever way they could, and so their English resources were stretched. Second, because they had no control over the BSL source they could not rely on their learnt writing structures that they used in the picture-based text (such as the repetition of character names). Thirdly, the influence of the BSL source may have inhibited the use of these strategies.

It is important to note that, contrary to the assumption made at the outset of this task, it emerged that the picture source was by no means 'language free'. This became apparent as the children all drew on and deployed their repertoire of set English phrases and structures associated with this reading scheme. It could be argued therefore that the picture-based text provided an indirect English source because of these associations. Despite this, we were able to draw some valid comparisons.

The unexpected finding from this analysis is that the children's picture-based texts were generally more correct but more repetitive and less complex than the translation texts. Although for most of the children there was not a marked difference in the length of their two texts, most of them attempted more complex grammatical sequences in their translation text than they did in their picture-based text. This is mainly evident though their use of simple and subordinate clauses and simple or complex noun phrases. This finding suggests that what the children have formally learnt about writing English (evident in their picture-based writing) is limited compared to their potential for more diverse and complex written expression.

Implications for literacy instruction

One of the basic tenets of bilingual education is that the more use is made of the learner's first language, the higher becomes the learner's proficiency in their second language. Within the field of sign bilingual education, ways of interpreting this are being explored that try to clarify the role of sign language in English learning and teaching and maximize the pupils established linguistic skills and resources.

From the preliminary analysis of the data provided by this study it emerged that unless the deaf pupils have strong spoken language skills the composing stage of their English writing relies more heavily on the application of their knowledge of BSL. Evidence from the wider field of bilingualism and literacy points to a need to harness this application or transfer of skills, since these strategies enable pupils to plan and compose independently.

For deaf pupils, given their specific linguistic situation, more emphasis needs to placed on the development of their awareness of the differences between BSL and written English so that they can begin to appreciate what they can appropriately apply from BSL to the writing task. For example, the children's approaches to the writing task in this study could have been further supported by discussion of the differences between 'live' story telling (as in the BSL source) and written narrative since many of the children tried to recreate the sense of 'live' in their writing that caused them problems regarding the use of definite and indefinite articles. Collaborative dialogue in L1 has been found to support other second-language learners by enabling them to collectively build knowledge about their L2 (Swain, 2000).

Alongside this support through discussion in sign language, deaf pupils also need plentiful exposure to the different conventions of written English through wide and guided reading activities. This implies a reading programme which aims to focuses the learner's attention on the structures and conventions of written English, in addition to developing their individual reading skills. Deaf children's early writing might then be further supported by the use of structured materials such as writing frames and models.

This dual focus of language awareness raising through sign language and exposure to writing conventions through text would aim to compensate for the lack of prior literacy experience and full access to spoken English. Recreating the conditions for emerging literacy development which is experienced by most hearing children, and on which bilingual hearing children are able to build, is not realistic for deaf children whose primary language is sign language. The goal instead should be to maximize the advantages deaf children's bilingualism affords. This entails building on their tacit knowledge of languages, resulting from their experience of constantly moving between the different conventions and modalities of BSL and English, and shaping this into a resource for their second-language learning.

Chapter 8
Promoting social and emotional development in deaf children: linking theory and practice

PETER HINDLEY

There is a growing body of evidence that promoting social and emotional functioning should be a core component of ensuring that deaf children achieve their academic potential (see Gray et al, 2001). Research with hearing children is demonstrating that good social and emotional functioning is strongly associated with academic achievement and that good social and emotional functioning is driven by key early experiences: promoting secure attachment relationships (Belsky and Cassidy, 1994) and providing pre-school children with experience of conversations about mental and emotional experience (Dunn, 1996). This direct experience of other people's emotional states appears to play a central role in the development and experience of empathy (Adolphs, 2002). There are reasons to believe that deaf children from hearing families (DH) are particularly at risk of delays and disorders of social and emotional development. Earlier studies have suggested that DH children tend to be more impulsive than hearing children, are more egocentric, have more restricted emotional vocabularies and more limited understanding of emotional processes and more limited social problems solving skills (Hindley, 2000).

In addition, DH children are more at risk of developing child mental health problems. The processes that lead to this increased risk are complex, but it appears likely that access to early communication and access to incidental learning are two of the key social processes that can promote resilience or, if they are absent or their increase is restricted, may increase the vulnerability DH children. Lack of or reduced access to early communication within the family will reduce DH's experience of conversations about emotions and mental states. This can be both direct (adults and other children talking to them) and indirect ('overhearing' conversations about emotions and mental states). The latter is one aspect of incidental learning – the chance, informal learning that is a key component of all children's developmental experience (Greenberg, 2000). DH children, particularly in mainstream educational settings, are likely to have reduced access to all aspects of incidental learning, but particularly social and emotional experiences which develop quickly and entail sophisticated and often implicit social interactions.

However, school may also be the setting in which many of these delays may be redressed (Greenberg, 2000). Early social and emotional experience at home is a key early driver of development. When children enter school, social and emotional interactions with children, teachers and other adults become equally important. Experience at school is probably even more important for deaf children than for hearing children. This is especially so for deaf children from families with limited communication skills. For these children interactions with deaf peers, teachers, other staff and hearing children with appropriate communication skills assume even greater importance developmentally. Even for children from high communication families, a sense of shared experience with other deaf children can mean that interactions with deaf peers have greater emotional resonance. When considering the school's role in addressing social and emotional delays in deaf children, a number of difficulties emerge:

- Most primary schools use curricular and pastoral activities that assume that children entering school do not have significant delays.
- In order to address these delays, deaf children need direct experience of social and emotional interactions that are explicitly linked to enhancing linguistic and cognitive skills. This is not always true for peer–peer interactions or informal interactions with adults.
- Much of the emphasis in schools in the western world, although not exclusively, is on academic achievement rather than social and emotional development. In order for schools to address these problems they need access to the means of artificially re-creating earlier developmental experience but at the same time meeting demands for academic targets (Greenberg, 2000).

There are a wide variety of interventions aimed at promoting the social or behavioural functioning of children in schools (see Greenberg, 2000 for a review). Two packages of school based interventions covering social, emotional behavioural functioning are currently in common use in the USA and, to a lesser extent, Great Britain. The Incredible Years (*http://www.incredibleyears.com*) and Promoting Alternative Thinking Strategies or PATHS (Greenberg and Kusché, 1993) are both used with primary school children. They both place considerable emphasis on building self-esteem, behavioural self-control and social problem-solving skills in children through direct classroom-based experiences led by teachers. The major difference between PATHS and The Incredible Years is that PATHS places greater emphasis on building children's understanding of emotional processes and relationships. Both make extensive use of role-play, both rely on a combination of teacher-led imparting of skills and teacher-facilitated structured group work. It is the latter's greater emphasis on emotional understanding that makes it particularly relevant to deaf children.

This chapter reviews the recent literature in relation to both social and emotional development in deaf children and interventions aimed at enhancing deaf children's development. A key concern has been the extent to which these school-based interventions generalize to home and out of school settings. Will children use social and emotional skills developed in the school setting in other settings, such as home? The chapter presents a re-analysis of data from an earlier study of the use of PATHS in British schools. The re-analysis focuses specifically on the extent to which the introduction of PATHS lead to changes in children's behaviour at home.

Deaf children: theory of mind and emotional development

Two areas of research activity are deepening our understanding of the developmental processes that can enhance the psychological resilience of deaf children: the development of theory of mind and emotional understanding in deaf children (Gray et al, 2001; Remmel, Bettger and Weinberg, 2001).

Theory of mind is a relatively recent psychological construct (Flavell and Miller, 1998) that describes the process by which children begin to understand that their understanding and experience of the world may or may not be the same as other people's. The three main domains of theory of mind are desires, appearance, and false belief.

- **Desires** describes children's understanding that other people have different desires than themselves – some people argue that the 'terrible twos' (that is, the difficult behaviour in many 2-year-olds) arise from this growing understanding.
- **Appearance** describes children's understanding that one thing may appear to be the same as another, e.g. a piece of sponge painted to look like a rock, and another person may be deceived by this illusion.
- **False beliefs** describes children's understanding that another person has a different set of beliefs about people than themselves, which may be wrong. The latter has been assessed using psychological tests such as the Sally Ann test. In this test a child observes a glove puppet, Sally Ann, putting an object in a toy basket and leaving the 'room'. Another glove puppet then comes in and moves the object to a box.

Children are asked to say where Sally Ann will look for the object when she returns. Children who have developed an understanding that other people will have different, false, beliefs that explain people's behaviour than themselves will say that Sally Ann will look in the basket because that is where Sally Ann left it. Sally Ann does not know that the object has been moved, unlike the child who witnessed the other glove puppet moving the object. Children who have not developed this understanding say that Sally Ann will look in the box because this is where they know that the object is but do not realize that Sally Ann does not know this.

There have been over a dozen research studies investigating this aspect of deaf children's development. There have been a number of concerns about the methods used, and particularly the linguistic demands involved (Peterson and Siegal, 1999) and findings are not consistent across all studies. However, the majority of studies suggest that DH children, when compared with DD children and hearing children are far more likely to show evidence of delays in developing theory of mind with respect to false beliefs but not with respect to desire and appearance (Gray et al, 2001; Remmel, Bettger and Weinberg, 2001). A conservative estimate would suggest that DH children are commonly 3–4 years behind their hearing peers in developing theory of mind (Lundy, 2002), only passing false belief tests, on average, at age 7–8 years. A more radical position would suggest that up to 70% of DH 7-year-olds will not pass false belief tests, the same being true for many DH teenagers. This compares with DD children (Courtin and Melot, 1998; Courtin, 2000) who will develop theory of mind at the same rate as hearing children of hearing parents, when factors such as social class are taken into account. That is, that by approximately 4–5 years of age, most understand that another person has a different set of beliefs than themselves. As Remmel, Bettger and Weinberg (2001) suggest, this implies that many DH children are operating using the desire psychology of 2- and 3-year-old hearing children. This should not be taken to mean that these delays affect deaf children's overall level of functioning, but rather that their performance can be patchy with key elements delayed and others age appropriate.

This can be seen in aspects of deaf children's understanding of emotion. Gray et al (2001) have shown that deaf children at ages 7 and 11 show the same abilities to recognize basic emotional expressions (happy, sad, angry, surprised, disgusted) and make similar mistakes, e.g. 7-year-old deaf and hearing children are more likely to identify happy, sad and angry but more likely to confuse disgusted with angry and surprised with happy. Deaf children show similar skills in understanding rules which govern overt displays of emotion or display rules. This is the process by which children begin to realize that there are social expectations linked to expressions of emotion – smiling and saying thank you when you receive a present, appearing sympathetic when somebody is upset – which may not reflect children's real feelings and help children to decide when and when not to express particular emotions. There is evidence that, for hearing children, the acquisition of display rules is related to overall levels of social maturity (Garner, 1996).

There appear to be similarities and differences in the way that DH and hearing children acquire display rules. Gray et al (2001) studied children's responses to signed and spoken social stories and found that 7- and 14-year old DH and hearing children both show evidence of using display rules but that there were differences in the kinds of emotions that they chose to conceal. DH and hearing children were just as likely to conceal emotions such as fear that might put them at risk of physical harm, but were less likely to hide emotions that might upset other people such as anger or expressions of happiness for pro-social reasons, i.e. to avoid upsetting another child when you have won something (95% of 7- and 14-year-old hearing children against 50% of 7-year-old and 70% of 14-year-old DH children; Gray et al, 2001:144).

Both of these sets of display rules are acquired through socialization. However, learning the importance of hiding one's own feelings in order to avoid hurting another person's feelings is a considerably more complex rule than learning to conceal feelings that might put one at risk of being hit by another child. The latter has clear and immediate benefits, whereas the benefits of the former will be delayed and expressed mainly through verbal interactions with friends and family. Gray et al (2001) have also suggested that some DH children show delays in experiencing and recognizing ambivalent or contradictory emotions, although their findings are less consistent in this area. However their suggestion is consistent with earlier findings (Greenberg and Kusché, 1993) that have shown that deaf children's vocabulary of emotions is often restricted and that their understanding of complex emotions such as jealousy or disappointment is often limited.

In summary, recent research on the social and emotional development of DH children suggests that there are significant delays in core elements of development, particularly with respect to an understanding of other people's thinking and emotions, for some but not all children. What factors lead to this developmental delay and what can we do to prevent or remediate them? There is less direct evidence here, but two major factors can be inferred. The first is that factors associated with the various causes of deafness are contributing to these social and emotional delays. A variety of aetiological factors are associated with disabilities of varying kinds. Those disorders and disabilities that are associated with pervasive brain disorders may explain why DH children are vulnerable to these social and emotional delays, akin but not identical to difficulties seen in hearing children with autism. On the other hand DH children are more vulnerable to a range of social risk factors.

They are more likely to have difficulties in communicating with their families than DD or HH children. In particular, their parents are more likely to simplify their language and less likely to talk about emotional and mental states because they lack the language to do so and DH children are more likely to have difficulty 'overhearing' conversations about such psychological states.

There is no direct evidence as to the relative importance of these two sets of factors and it is likely that in reality they interact, but a range of factors suggest that social risk factors are more significant.

- First, the studies of theory of mind have used non-verbal measures of intelligence to ensure that the children's delays could not be accounted for by general cognitive delays.
- Second, one study has used a measure of language development in the DH children, which ensured that they were matched for BSL development with their DD controls and yet still showed highly significant delays in their development of theory of mind (Woolfe, Want and Siegal, 2002).
- Third, the proportion of deaf children with causes of deafness associated with brain disorders accounts for only 30% of DH children, and not all of these will have significant brain disorders; only some 15% (Freeman, Malkin and Hastings, 1975) have neurological signs of brain disorders, when some studies report up 70% of DH children showing significant delays in theory of mind.
- Fourth, DH children show the capacity to develop understanding of emotional states and pro-social skills linked to theory of mind when provided the appropriate intervention (Greenberg and Kusché, 1993; Hindley and Reed, 1999; and below) which suggests that these delays are the result of deprivation of experience rather than difficulties in processing social and psychological information as a result of subtle brain disorders.

It is important to reiterate that not all DH children will be vulnerable to these developmental delays. However, those that are affected by delays in the development of theory of mind and various aspects of emotional functioning are likely to be more vulnerable to various child mental health problems. Children who function on a desire psychology, to simplify grossly, children who understand that other people want different things from them but do not understand why, are likely to be at greater risk of behavioural problems. Whenever they encounter a situation where they want to do something and the other person does not want them to, or vice versa, they will not have access to the buffering effect of understanding why the other person does or does not want them to do something. Additionally, they are likely to have greater difficulty in understanding the other person's reasoning.

Hindley and Reed (1999) were able to demonstrate significant changes in emotional understanding and improved social functioning in the school setting among 8–10-year-old deaf children exposed to PATHS. This chapter presents additional data examining the impact of PATHS on parent rated social and emotional adjustment.

The study

The original study is described in greater detail in Hindley and Reed (1999). It used a waiting-list design to assess the effectiveness of PATHS in British primary schools. The study divided the schools involved into two groups. One group received the intervention at the beginning of the project (T0). The other group did not receive any intervention for the first year, thus acting as a 'waiting list' control group. The analysis focused on differences between the two groups in the rates of change of children's scores on measures used over the first year of the project. And the extent to which any differences in rates of change altered after the waiting list group received the intervention at 1 year (T2). All children had baseline assessments of social, emotional and cognitive functioning prior to the introduction of PATHS (T0), Group 1 then received the curriculum. All of the children were reassessed at 6 months (T1). The children were reassessed at 12 months (T2), just before Group 2 received the curriculum, and the children were re-assessed again at 21 months, the end of the study. The main outcome measure was a comparison of the two groups' rate of development across different developmental domains over the first year of the study.

PATHS is a social and emotional curriculum designed specifically to enhance the social and emotional development of deaf children. It consists of over 100 lessons, divided into three sections: Readiness and Self-Control; Feelings and Relationships: and Problem-solving. Throughout the curriculum is designed to enhance four domains of functioning:

- **affective:** recognition and understanding of one's own and other's emotions
- **behaviour:** a capacity to monitor and control one's own behaviour
- **cognitive:** developing skills to recognize and solve social problems
- **dynamic:** an understanding of relationships (Greenberg and Kusché, 1993).

The curriculum places greater emphasis on different aspects at different stages, with the intent of mirroring the normal sequence of social and emotional development.

The Readiness and Self-Control section concentrates on developing behavioural control and enhancing self-esteem. The former is achieved by the use of the Turtle Technique, introduced to the children by a moral fable about a little tortoise (or turtle in North American English) who cannot control himself but learns to do so after being taught by a wise old tortoise. The essential components are to: stop, say what the problem is and say how you are feeling. This internal process is demonstrated externally by specific behaviours that child displays and that the teacher can reinforce. It is supported by the use of traffic light and turtle motifs throughout the school. These external behaviours can later be faded out and replaced by purely cognitive processes but re-activated if the child needs greater support. The Turtle Technique thus introduces the child to basic problem-solving techniques.

The use of the story allows the teacher to introduce the theory and practice of role-play in a non-threatening way. Role-play will later become an essential part of the curriculum. The component of the first unit that aims to enhance self-esteem is a combination of a teacher's assistant, the PATHS 'child for the day' and the giving of compliments. The PATHS child for the day not only helps the teacher during PATHS time but also receives compliments from his or her classmates. Research into the development of empathy (see above) supports the anecdotal observation that children's growing sophistication in this process underpins many aspects of pro-social behaviour. Thus early on the children tended to compliment each other on their possessions or physical characteristics (trainers, hair, etc.), as the curriculum progressed they began to compliment each other for behaviour such as helping each other in the playground or with homework. This capacity to recognize pro-social behaviour in others appeared to reflect the development of a greater capacity to empathize with others.

The Feelings and Relationships Unit concentrates on developing emotional understanding and understanding of relationships. The components of the first unit are maintained but a range of emotions are introduced in lessons that use stories and games to explain the meaning of each of the emotions. This is supported by the use of Emotions Cards that show the facial expression of a particular emotion and the English word. The unit starts with basic emotions such as happy, sad and surprised but develops to include emotions such as jealous, disappointed and malicious. At the same time the meaning of emotions and their role in human relationships are explored by the use of increasingly sophisticated and challenging role-plays. However, because role-play has been introduced early and in a non-threatening way, the children and teacher have sufficient confidence in their technique and the group to explore and experience difficult feelings such as jealousy. As the second unit progresses it moves from scripted stories about feelings and relationships to stories that the children themselves generate and the teacher begins to introduce to the skills involved in social problem-solving.

The third component concentrates on social problem-solving in a structured and increasingly sophisticated way. The aim of the Unit is to help the children develop consequential thinking skills rather than goal-oriented thinking skills. That is, thinking skills that not only enable children to achieve their goals but to anticipate what the consequences of their plan is and evaluate the consequences of a number of different plans. This is initially taught in a formal way using an 11-step problem-solving approach. The skills are initially taught using scripted problems and exercises but increasingly children are encouraged to put forward everyday life problems. Problems are discussed and solved in problem-solving groups that emphasize group interaction and sharing of different perspectives. In the study the problems ranged from mundane but essential, problems such as how to share a football at lunchtime to how to solve the problems of the Middle East. Where problems impact on the wider school system, people from outside the class are encouraged to join the class in discussing and solving the problems.

The aim of the curriculum is to provide both direct experience of a social and emotional interaction and the skills (linguistic, cognitive, social and emotional) to use this experience in all parts of the child's life. The curriculum employs a wide range of teaching techniques and significantly enhances vocabularies, especially of emotions, but central is the use of role-play, initially in a carefully prescribed way but later to reconstruct real life problems. There is a strong emphasis on creating, albeit artificially, normal developmental experience.

PATHS is intentionally focused on the school environment, and in the main it has been used by teachers with additional training. In one British study the curriculum has been delivered by primary child mental health workers, working alongside teachers, as part of a primary child mental health intervention. There are elements throughout the curriculum that link school and home activities. However, the deliberate emphasis is on the school, with the aim of not overburdening deaf children's parents with additional work. Rather home–school activities are aimed at keeping parents informed of developments at school and on ensuring that parents are aware of new vocabulary – either signed or spoken – that the children are being introduced to. The schools involved in the study were scattered over a wide geographical area and half were residential schools. The study used intensive family weekends to enhance the parent involvement in the intervention and target specific areas such as the parents' behaviour management skills, feelings about becoming parents of deaf children and sibling relationships (NDCS, 1999).

Given that the predominant focus was on the school environment, how much change can be expected to take place in the home environment? This criticism has been levelled at a range of school-based interventions such social skills training or purely behavioural interventions (see Greenberg, 2000) where changes often do not generalize from school to home. One of the aims of PATHS is to integrate social, emotional and cognitive change with linguistic and dynamic development. Can we expect that PATHS will lead to more generalizable developmental change that can be seen at home? It was with this in mind that the data was re-analysed.

Re-analysis: aims

The re-analysis examined the effect of the intervention on the social adjustment of both groups of children involved in the study, as assessed by parents. It differed from the original analysis in using a before-and-after measure combined for both groups, and not the waiting list design of the original study. The aims of the re-analysis were to examine whether or not the intervention had lead to any change in social functioning at home. One of the major criticisms of many interventions aimed at enhancing children's social and emotional functioning is that they are context-dependent. That is, that they may lead to significant change in the context within which the intervention is delivered, but not in other domains of the children's lives. If this held true for the use of PATHS in this study no change would be observed in the other area of the children's lives at home.

Subjects

The children involved in the study were all children with severe to profound sensorineural deafness, aged 7–11. They attended four schools for deaf children and three hearing impaired units attached to mainstream schools. Since this was a school-based project, most of the contact with children was in school and contact with parents was via schools, except for those families who attended the two family weekends – approximately one-fifth of the group. There were 63 children in the study, of whom 31 completed parental measures at the beginning of the study and 22 at the end of the study, 2 years later. The fact that most of the contact was indirect may partly account for the high attrition rate in the final follow-up.

Method

Pre-, intra- and post- intervention measures were administered to the children. All children received a full academic year of PATHS, delivered by teachers who had received specific training in the use of PATHS. The curriculum was delivered in different ways in each of the schools. All schools were advised to provide a full lesson of PATHS a minimum of 4 days/week. However the demands of the National Curriculum meant that some schools were only able to deliver 3 lessons/week. Teachers paced the delivery of the curriculum according to the needs of their pupils and all schools were able to deliver the full curriculum over the academic year.

The original study was designed as a waiting list control intervention, with one group receiving the intervention in the first year, while the other group waited a year before receiving the intervention. In this re-analysis the groups have been merged and change before and after intervention has been measured, i.e. between T0 and T3.

Measures

The original study used a wide variety of measures, administered to children, teachers and parents (see Hindley and Reed, 1999 for details). The re-analysis concerned one measure, the parents' Strengths and Difficulties Questionnaire (SDQ). This is a 25-item behavioural questionnaire which exists in parent, teacher and self-report formats. It has been widely used amongst hearing children (e.g. Goodman, Meltzer and Bailey, 1998) and has good validity and reliability properties. It has particularly good user satisfaction properties since it is relatively short and contains both positive and negative behavioural items. It was selected for this reason, even though at the time of the study it was not validated with deaf children. However, there are no items related to spoken language and for this reason it appeared to have face validity. Further information concerning the SDQ can be found in Goodman, Meltzer and Bailey (1998).

Parents are asked to consider their child's behaviour over the previous 6 months and indicate whether each behavioural item is: not true; somewhat true; or certainly true.

The SDQ total score, can be used but factor analysis has found that specific items group into specific scales: pro-social, conduct problems, emotional symptoms, hyperactivity and peer-problems. In all cases, including the pro-social scale, higher scores reflect higher rates of problems. The specific behavioural items for each of the subscales are as follows:

- **Pro-social scale:** Considerate of other people's feelings; shares readily with other children (treats, toys, pencils, etc.); helpful if someone is hurt, upset or feeling ill; kind to younger children; often volunteers to help others (parents, teachers, other children).
- **Hyperactivity scale:** Restless, overactive, cannot stay still for long; constantly fidgeting or squirming; easily distracted, concentration wanders; thinks things out before acting; sees tasks through to the end, good attention span.
- **Conduct problems scale:** Often has temper tantrums or hot tempers; generally obedient, usually does what adults request; often fights with other children or bullies them; often lies or cheats; steals things from home, school or elsewhere.

- **Emotional symptoms scale:** Often complains of headaches, stomach-aches or sickness; many worries, often seems worried; often unhappy, downhearted or tearful; nervous or clingy in new situations, easily loses confidence; many fears, easily scared.
- **Peer problems scale:** Rather solitary, tends to play alone; has at least one good friend; generally liked by other children; picked on or bullied by other children; gets on better with adults than with other children.

Results

Data was missing on 8 of the 63 children. There were 34 boys and 21 girls (62% vs 38%); 39 of the children attended schools for deaf children and 16 attended hearing impaired units. Their mean age at the start of the study was 8.9 years.

Thirty-one parents completed the SDQ at the beginning of the study and 22 at the end. Eighteen parents completed SDQs at the beginning and the end. Mean SDQ total and scale scores are shown in Table 8.1.

Table 8.1 Mean total and scale SDQ scores

	N	Minimum	Maximum	Mean	SD
TOT0	31	13.00	34.00	22.6774	5.7410
TOT3	22	6.00	34.00	19.0455	7.6499
PS0	31	4.00	10.00	7.3226	1.4233
PS3	22	0.00	10.00	5.5217	3.0581
ES0	31	0.00	10.00	3.1613	2.5311
ES3	22	1.00	6.00	3.4783	1.7547
HS0	31	0.00	8.00	4.0968	2.3431
HS3	22	1.00	8.00	4.5909	2.0623
CS0	31	1.00	8.00	3.9677	1.7026
CS3	22	0.00	7.00	3.1364	2.0998
PP0	31	2.00	8.00	4.1290	1.8751
PP3	22	0.00	6.00	2.4545	1.6826
Valid N (listwise)	18				

Tot+total; PS, pro-social; ES, emotional symptoms; HS, hyperactivity; CS, conduct; PP, peer problems; SD, standard deviation

The mean total scores, pro-social, conduct and peer-problem scale scores fell for the whole group over the 2-year intervention period. The mean emotional symptom and hyperactivity scale scores rose over the same period.

In order to assess the significance of change during the intervention, paired *t*-tests were performed on the 18 SDQs completed at the beginning and end of the study. A greater proportion of the paired group attended deaf schools (15/18 vs 39/55 or 83% vs. 71%), there was a greater proportion of boys (78%) and the mean age of the children in the paired group was slightly lower at 8.7%.

These mean total and scale scores of these 18 children are shown in Table 8.2 and the paired t-tests are shown in Table 8.3.

Table 8.2 Paired samples mean total and scale SDQ scores

		Mean	N	SD	SME
Pair 1	TOT0	25.0000	18	5.2692	1.2420
	TOT3	17.1667	18	6.9557	1.6395
Pair 2	PS0	7.6316	18	1.1648	0.2672
	PS3	5.1053	18	3.0349	0.6963
Pair 3	ES0	3.9474	18	2.5922	0.5947
	ES3	3.1579	18	1.7405	0.3993
Pair 4	HS0	4.5556	18	2.1205	0.4998
	HS3	4.2778	18	2.0236	0.4770
Pair 5	CS0	4.2778	18	1.6017	0.3775
	CS3	2.5000	18	1.6539	0.3898
Pair 6	PP0	4.4444	18	1.9166	0.4517
	PP3	2.3333	18	1.6803	0.3961

SD, standard deviation; SME, standard error of the mean.

As with the whole group mean total scores, pro-social, conduct and peer problem scale scores fell in the paired group. In contrast to the whole group both mean emotional symptom and hyperactivity scales also fell following the intervention in the paired group.

Table 8.3 Paired samples test total and scale SDQ scores

		Paired differences	SD	SME	95% Confidence interval of the difference		t	df	Sig. (2-tailed)
		Mean			Lower	Upper			
Pair 1	TOT0–TOT3	7.8333	7.6100	1.7937	4.0490	11.6177	4.367	17	0.000
Pair 2	PS0–PS3	2.5263	2.9130	0.6683	1.1223	3.9303	3.780	17	0.001
Pair 3	ES0–ES3	0.7895	3.1016	0.7116	-0.7054	2.2844	1.110	17	0.282
Pair 4	HS0–HS3	0.2778	2.8244	0.6657	-1.1268	1.6823	0.417	17	0.682
Pair 5	CS0–CS3	1.7778	1.8960	0.4469	0.8349	2.7206	3.978	17	0.001
Pair 6	PP0–PP3	2.1111	1.6047	0.3782	1.3131	2.9091	5.581	17	0.000

SD, standard deviation; SME, standard error of the mean

However, paired t-tests revealed that only the changes in the total scores, pro-social, conduct and peer problem scale scores were statistically significantly.

Discussion

These findings suggest that the positive effects of PATHS on deaf children's social and emotional development in school, found in the original study, generalized to their home environments. However, there are weaknesses in this study. Only 56% of parents completed SDQs at the beginning of the study, 40% at the end and 33% at both beginning and end. Children who benefited from the intervention may be over-represented in this sample and this may explain the positive result. However, the children's mean age was almost identical to that of the overall study group. In addition, the subgroup's sex and schooling characteristics are both associated with greater risks of social and emotional delays and problems. There is substantial evidence that girls show greater social maturity than boys and that boys are more vulnerable to child mental health problems that would be identified by an instrument such as the SDQ. In addition, children with additional social and emotional needs tend to be over-represented in schools for deaf children, and particularly residential schools. On the other hand it is possible that the greater curricular flexibility, and overall control over the school environment, at the schools for deaf children meant that they could deliver PATHS more effectively and reinforce its components more effectively during and after school.

A further area of concern is the ability of hearing parents to rate the behaviour and emotions of DH children. Lack of conversational experience about emotions has already been cited as one possible mechanism for developmental delay. How able are hearing parents assess their children's emotional states if they do not have sufficient vocabulary? Studies of clinical populations of deaf children with mental health problems suggest that children with emotional disorders are not identified by parents or teachers (Hindley and van Gent, 2000). Equally there is evidence that communication between some DH children and young people and their parents can be extremely limited (Gregory, Bishop and Sheldon, 1995). This may cast some doubt on some hearing parents' ability to accurately assess their DH children's emotional states.

If the results are reliable, the more detailed scale results are of considerable interest. The significant improvements in both pro-social and peer problem scores suggest that PATHS is positively affecting the areas of social and emotional delays which it explicitly targets. These findings are reinforced by recent research suggesting that delays in emotional understanding in deaf children can particularly affect subtle pro-social skills (Gray et al, 2001). They also throw light on widely reported peer-relationship difficulties amongst deaf children (see Hindley, 2000), by inference suggesting that these difficulties may in part arise from social skills deficits. The changes in the conduct scale are consistent with findings amongst hearing children with conduct problems. Studies of the social understanding of hearing children with conduct disorder suggest that deficits in pro-social skills contribute to their peer interaction problems (Happé and Frith, 1996).

It is of equal interest to note that although the children's emotional symptom scale scores fell, these changes were not statistically significant. The emotional symptom scale screens for a variety of emotional disorders that are affected by factors such as self-esteem and peer support. Self-esteem is specifically targeted by PATHS and the fall in the peer problem scale scores suggests, by inference, that peer support improves. It is therefore puzzling that PATHS, in this sample, has not had a statistically significant impact on emotional symptom scale scores.

The findings of this study suggest that an intervention such as PATHS can have a significant, positive impact on the social and emotional development DH children at school and at home. This is clearly of importance for parents of DH children who frequently have concerns about their children's emotional wellbeing. Such improvements are likely to have a significant impact on the quality of life of these families. However, the findings also have important implications for educators of deaf children and policy-makers. Enhancing deaf children's social and emotional development has immediate, medium and long-term effects. In the immediate term, teachers and parents are likely to see significant changes in pro-social behaviour with consequent positive impacts on class room atmosphere and attitudes towards learning. In the medium term, these changes should be associated with improving academic achievement but, equally importantly, positive changes in social behaviour and relationships with peers and adults. In the long term, interventions such as PATHS will play an important part in developing deaf children's skills and attitudes as future citizens and so enhancing deaf people's opportunities to play as full a part as possible in civic societies.

However, it is essential to note that for these long-term effects to be realized, interventions focused on middle childhood will not be sufficient. All of the social risk factors identified in the introduction to this chapter continue into adolescence, and continuing efforts will be required to maximize deaf children's social and emotional experience throughout their school years. All of this echoes the thoughts of many people in education, particularly parents, teachers and deaf adults. There will need to be a fundamental shift in education policy: a shift away from a vision of children as receptacles into which knowledge and skills can be poured and towards a vision of children as human beings who need the right environment, sometimes enriched, in order to grow into fully competent adults.

PART III
SUPPORT FOR LEARNING

Commentary

ALYS YOUNG AND CLARE GALLAWAY

Research linked to support for learning for deaf children or students faces many new and exciting challenges as it attempts to capture and understand a rapidly changing context. The fast pace of current technological innovation is creating new learning possibilities for children and changed expectations of achievement. Concepts of 'access' to education are broadening to encompass and emphasize the language preferences of those being educated and the duty of organizations to meet those preferences. Professionals working within educational settings are discovering new facets to their roles in light of the changes in learning support available to deaf children and students. The chapters in this section are reflective of these trends. Archbold and Nikolopoulos (Chapter 9) consider the impact of the rise in paediatric cochlear implantation on both the educational outcomes for deaf children and the role of professionals working in education. McCracken (Chapter 10) evaluates the potential gain within the educational setting from a two-channel compression hearing aid, from the perspectives of both deaf children and teachers. O'Neill and Laidler (Chapter 11) investigate the differences and suitability of three systems of text support available to deaf students in further education. Traynor and Harrington (Chapter 12) focus on BSL/English interpreting in higher education institutions and consider whether and how it provides access to the university curriculum.

Although the research projects reported vary in age of children considered, educational setting, and approach to language, three themes emerge that are consistent to all. They are an attention to 'evidence in context'; participatory methodologies; and a critical questioning of criteria by which outcomes should be defined.

With regard to evidence in context, McCracken and Archbold, in particular, are constantly mindful that evidence to support the advantages of a new technology – be it in hearing aids or cochlear implantation – means little unless those results can be generated and validated within the real-life contexts in which deaf children find themselves. The challenge is to create research methodologies that enable such evaluation to happen in the demanding conditions of a busy and active child's life and in the concentrated conditions of a child's experience of more formal educational settings. Similarly with regard to the effectiveness of text support and BSL/English interpreting, the potential of these approaches for improved linguistic access to the curriculum for deaf students is of less concern than the enactment of that potential within the educational context. The physical and attitudinal barriers to effective interpreting and the influence of the operator rather than simply the text system itself are key examples of the significance of context considered in these research studies.

In many respects, participatory methodologies in educational research with deaf children or students are in their infancy. But the chapters in this section do begin to question whether and how the views of deaf children or students should not just be considered within the research but actually come to guide the research design itself. As end users of a means of support, O'Neill and Laidler focus on individual preferences of deaf students for particular text systems, where individual preference is not linked in any straightforward way to the hearing or communication profile of the students themselves. McCracken explores the role of deaf children as active participants in evaluative research designs in a field in which it is surprisingly rare to ask child hearing-aid users about their experiences.

Finally, not only appropriate outcome measures, but appropriate criteria by which to consider outcomes, are a constant concern of these research studies. This is perhaps not surprising. Within the history of the education of deaf children in the UK, outcome has always been a rather contentious subject. Historically child communication, and in particular speech, were often viewed as key markers of a successful 'educational' experience rather than education per se. In the research covered in these chapters, approaches to outcome criteria employed include: enhanced linguistic ability, access to educational content, satisfaction with support system, usability of technology and degree of participation in educational experience. All are reflective of significant and complementary aspects of learning.

These linked concerns of evidence in context, participatory methodology and outcome criteria reflect the increasing awareness of the methodological challenges faced in attempting to gain a holistic understanding of the educational experience and needs of deaf children and students today. The diversity of focus of chapters in this section is indicative of the breadth with which researchers are now defining and engaging with the notion of learning support for deaf children and students.

Chapter 9
Multidisciplinary working practice: examples of research into outcomes from paediatric cochlear implantation

SUE ARCHBOLD AND THOMAS NIKOLOPOULOS

The introduction of paediatric cochlear implantation to the UK in 1989 brought a challenging new dimension to the management of profoundly deaf young children, with, then unthought of, implications for the education of the deaf. At that time, amid much controversy, only those children with vibro-tactile aided thresholds and with acquired losses were considered candidates for implantation. Expectations were very conservative: the provision of useful responses to environmental sounds and an aid to lip-reading. Since then, the outcomes from implantation have grossly exceeded these expectations, and, as a consequence, children with much greater levels of residual hearing are now receiving implants. Twelve years on, the implications of implantation in young, congenitally deaf children are only just becoming apparent, as larger numbers of children have been implanted over longer periods of time. The opportunities offered by implantation have also brought challenges for educators of the deaf, as the dramatic changes in expectation for some young deaf children have become clear, and, with them, their changing educational needs.

What changes in candidature have we seen over this period?

- more born-deaf children than those with acquired losses
- changes in audiological criteria, as those with implants outperform those with some residual hearing using conventional aids
- increasingly young children being implanted, including those in the first year of life
- older teenagers choosing to have implants for themselves

- more complex children receiving implants
- some deaf parents of deaf children now choosing implants for their child.

On what basis are these changes being made? Are they evidence-based? Paediatric cochlear implantation has not been without its critics (Lane and Bahan, 1998) and remains controversial for some. It is an elective operation and one which will change communication and educational choices for the deaf child; it also is an expensive option, both in the short term and the long term. It is therefore vital that the changes in criteria and the decisions made on behalf of young deaf infants should be evidence-led and that research and audit should form part of any clinical cochlear implant programme. Cochlear implantation is a medical and surgical procedure, with associated risks. Parents making the decision on behalf of their child must receive accurate, up-to-date information on the potential risks, and likely benefits and outcomes in order to make an informed decision. Frequently their child's Teacher of the Deaf (ToD) will be the person with whom they will discuss these issues; the ToD thus has a responsibility to be familiar with up-to-date technology, criteria and expected range of outcomes. Research and audit carried out by the cochlear implant centre must therefore be accessible, understandable and constantly reviewed.

Paediatric implantation involves an unusual number of professional disciplines working together as a team, and this chapter will review research carried out at the Nottingham Paediatric Cochlear Implant Programme in a number of areas, including audiological, medical, linguistic, educational and psycho-social.

Complex issues

Outcomes from cochlear implantation may be defined differently by parents, purchasers, professionals, representatives of the deaf community, and the children themselves as they grow up. Progress for any deaf child is influenced by a number of factors, including age at onset, aetiology, residual hearing, cognition, the presence of other learning difficulties and management. In the case of those with implants, progress is additionally influenced by other factors such as the functioning and tuning of the implant system, numbers of electrodes inserted, the age of fitting, length of usage and the device itself. These variables and their interactions pose challenges to those endeavouring to carry out rigorous research and audit, and to predict benefit. In addition, when looking at children with implants, benefit develops over years rather than months, and during this time the technology itself has changed, and the groups considered for implantation have changed. Thus one is measuring outcomes in changing populations using constantly changing technology, complicating analysis and making the drawing of robust conclusions difficult.

In research, the purists would argue for the use of randomized controlled trials to provide the evidence, but these have their difficulties. The selection procedures for such trials may make the subjects unrepresentative of the population from which they are drawn, and obtaining informed consent almost impossible. The rigorous conditions for such studies may well not reflect everyday life and routine clinical practice. In addition, as outlined above, the fast-moving technology and time taken to carry out such studies are likely to make the original research question redundant by the time long-term outcomes on significant numbers are obtained.

In spite of these challenges, the responsibility rests with cochlear implant teams to provide such information. Cochlear implant teams are unusual in the range of professionals they employ, including surgeons, scientists, radiologists, nursing staff, educators, speech and language therapists and psychologists. A specialist database is required which gathers data in all these areas, in order to explore relationships between them and to provide robust evidence to inform practice. This involves an unusual shared understanding and ownership of the data, and should involve those supporting the child at home and school rather than solely those at the implant clinic.

Medical and educational worlds

Although paediatric implantation involves such a range of professionals, it has brought together two professions more closely than ever before: surgeons and educators of the deaf. Clearly, implantation is a surgical procedure and one that was initially medically led. Why then, should educators of the deaf become closely involved?

In providing such useful hearing to profoundly deaf children, with typical aided thresholds following implantation of 35 dB(A) at 2 and 4 kHz (Nottingham Paediatric Cochlear Implant Programme Brochure), and enabling totally or profoundly deaf children to function as less deaf (Nakisa et al, 2001), there are implications for educators. Current generally accepted audiological criteria are losses greater than 105 dB, particularly in the high frequencies. These children have little or no useful hearing before implantation, and after implantation should be able to process spoken language via audition through the implant system. It follows that appropriate management is likely to change and that expectations are likely to change, bringing consequent challenges for ToDs.

Among the many challenges is the scrutiny of the education of the deaf by other professionals, who may have differing priorities. A survey of the most common problems faced by European cochlear implant centres (Archbold and Robinson, 1997) raised educational support as a major issue for coordinators of cochlear implant programmes.

Several studies attempt to link the educational management of deaf children with outcomes from cochlear implantation, and studies of the cost-effectiveness of the intervention are also scrutinizing educational management. Neither issue is straightforward, but they have brought the education of the deaf under the scrutiny of other professions. There arise several possible tensions between educators and cochlear implant centres:

- inequity of support between children with cochlear implants and those with hearing aids
- inequity of financial support
- differing expectations: cochlear implant clinic, parents, educators
- cochlear implantation may be intrusive in terms of family and educational time (Archbold and Robinson, 1997).

Some consider that cochlear implantation has directed resources away from other deaf children and their services, although it can be argued that all profoundly deaf children should be receiving the appropriate support they require, and it may well be that children with cochlear implants require less support in the long term. In addition, the ToD may be seen to have a large degree of responsibility for the outcomes from cochlear implantation, yet may not have been involved in the decision making, or the process itself. This can give rise to extra tensions for the ToDs closely involved in the management of those with cochlear implants, who may not have supported the decision to proceed.

In order to provide close liaison with those teachers working with children with cochlear implants, many implant centres in the UK have developed educational outreach programmes. ToDs based at the implant centre provide direct contact with the local service, and the responsibility for the children clearly rests with the local service and the implant centre provides the implant expertise and support. Local ToDs are involved from the outset in the assessment process and receive up-to-date information from the implant centre.

Which areas of research and audit are of interest to educators of the deaf?

With the introduction of newborn hearing screening in the UK, and early implantation becoming an increasing option, it is likely that in the near future the majority of profoundly deaf infants will receive implants. For ToDs, there are tremendous implications. Their role in the support of families following diagnosis will inevitably mean that they will be placed in the position of needing up-to-date information about referral criteria and procedures. For example, we know that early implantation leads to significantly better outcomes in terms of speech perception and production and differences in educational placement; misinformation may lead to delayed referrals and appropriate decisions being made. Parents have a right to accurate information on which to base their decision and, in many cases, it will be the ToD who is required to provide it.

Teachers of the deaf are also likely to be the ones to provide long-term support and management to both family and child. Practice should be informed by evidence and by the most recent research outcomes.

This chapter will give examples of the range of outcomes data from the Nottingham Paediatric Cochlear Implant Programme multidisciplinary database in the areas most pertinent to ToDs:

- usage rates
- surgical outcomes
- functioning and device problems
- speech perception and production
- linguistic outcomes
- educational decisions
- influences on outcomes
- psycho-social issues
- educational attainments
- employment outcomes.

Usage rates after implantation

Whether children continue to wear their implant systems may well be a good indicator of benefit; unlike other implantable devices, they have the choice as to whether to wear their system or not, and can switch off the external system. Some reports of high non-use rates (Rose, Vernon and Pool, 1996) led to Nottingham implant programme looking at its non-use rate (Archbold, Lutman and Nikolopoulos, 1998). At that time there were no non-users; since then, the non-use rate has varied between 1 and 2%, depending at which interval one takes the figures. They remain low (Figure 9.1), however, and relate to age at implant and attendance at a school for the deaf.

Surgical outcomes

Audit data currently informs that, with over 300 children implanted, the complication rate remains low. In 300 consecutively implanted children there were no major perioperative complications (within 1 day after

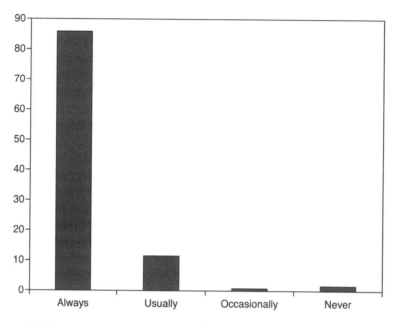

Figure 9.1 The use of the device 5 years after implantation, according to parents.

surgery) or major early postoperative complications (within 1 week after surgery). In the same periods there were 26 and 17 minor complications respectively (one child could have more than one complication). These complications settled with conservative treatment or minor intervention. There were 10 major late surgical complications (over 1 week after surgery) requiring re-operation or explantation (3 cases) and 20 minor (mild flap infection, flap swelling, etc.). There were also 10 cases of device failures that were all successfully re-implanted. In conclusion, cochlear implantation is a safe surgical operation in experienced centres. Most surgical complications are minor and can be managed with conservative treatment or minor surgical intervention.

Functioning of the device

The professionals of the cochlear implant team need to assess if the device is working, appropriately tuned for that child and providing benefit. For ToDs working with young deaf infants, and unable to listen to the implant functioning itself, it is important that, even with the youngest child, there are opportunities to monitor device functioning. Long-term research and audit will then enable the teacher to be aware if there are any significant difficulties with a particular child compared to the group data.

Apart from electrophysiological and technical testing that may reveal problems in the device function, steady progress in outcome measures gives reassurance that the cochlear implant system works properly and management is effective. Numerous device malfunctions have been suspected by ToDs because of a decrease or plateau in the rate of children's progress. Most of these malfunctions were subsequently confirmed by electrophysiological testing.

One measure which has been found useful with young infants is the Listening Progress Profile (LiP). This measure has been shown to be repeatable across users (Archbold, 1994). One study of early auditory performance using LiP in 68 young implanted children illustrates its use. Half of the children performing at or below the 10th percentile at the 1 year interval after implantation were later found to have device problems, and were subsequently re-implanted. Only 3% of the children performing above the 10th percentile of LiP were subsequently re-implanted (Nikolopoulos, Wells and Archbold, 2000).

Communication development

With young infants, the provision of useful hearing can be influential in the development of early communication skills, the precursors of language development. How can we measure this? Tait video analysis is a quantitative methodology for assessing preverbal communication skills in children with hearing aids and cochlear implants (Tait, Lutman and Nikolopoulos, 2001). It is shown to be reliable and free from observer bias (Tait, Nikolopoulos, Lutman, Wilson and Wells, 2001). Profoundly deaf young children, either with cochlear implants or successful users of hearing aids, show similar patterns of preverbal communication development that contrast with those of unsuccessful hearing-aid users. Pre-implant children's autonomy as measured by Tait video-analysis has been found to correlate significantly with closed-set tests (Iowa Matrix test) and open-set tests (Connected Discourse Tracking) at the 3-year interval after implantation, accounting for up to a quarter of the variance (Tait, Lutman, and Robinson, 2000). This is a noteworthy figure when studies of speech perception in general and cochlear implantation in particular are notorious for unexplained variance (O'Donoghue, Nikolopoulos and Archbold, 2000).

Difficulties in measuring speech perception and production

Before implantation, children are unlikely to have access to the entire speech signal and the major aim of implantation is to provide useful hearing across the speech frequencies. However, assessing progress in this area extends over a long time frame which may be 5 years or more.

Numerous studies in the literature (more than 600 articles up to the end of the year 2001) have investigated the various aspects of speech perception and speech production following cochlear implantation. The following three examples illustrate the difficulties in the respective research.

- Miyamoto et al (1995) studied 24 prelingually deaf children and found that cochlear implant children outperformed in speech perception the 'silver' hearing aid users (unaided thresholds between 101 and 110 dB at two of the three frequencies; 500, 1000 and 2000 Hz). Their performance was similar to that of 'gold' hearing users (unaided thresholds between 90 and 100 dB at two of the three frequencies; 500, 1000 and 2000 Hz). Although this study was a benchmark for cochlear implantation, some of the subjects entered the study after implantation and some intervals were combined to have more data.
- Waltzmann et al (1997) explored the open-set speech perception abilities of congenitally deaf children after cochlear implantation. Although this was a rather homogenous group, the numbers ranged from 38 evaluable children at the 1-year interval down to 3 children at 5 years. Accepting the declining sample size with the passage of time, their results were very encouraging: on the Glendonald Auditory Screening Procedure word test, the mean scores were 92%, 86% and 94% correct at the 3-, 4- and 5-year intervals after implantation. Similarly, on the PBK word test, their scores were 44%, 33% and 58% over the same periods (chance score 0% on both these tests).
- Moog and Geers (1999) reported that almost half of the children studied demonstrated language skills after implantation in the average range when compared to normal-hearing children their age, and that the vast majority of the children had excellent speech intelligibility. In spite of the rather thorough design of the study, the 22 participants were children attending the same oral school with length of implant use ranging widely from 1 to 7 years without giving data in specific intervals. Pre-implant performance was not included in some of the tests used, and there were no other important demographic details of the children such as aetiology of deafness, age at onset of deafness and whether postlingually deafened children were included.

Interpretation of the vast majority of the studies assessing speech perception and production after cochlear implantation is compromised by the use of soft outcome measures that have not been validated, the inclusion of children of widely differing ages and linguistic abilities, the retrospective nature of the data, small sample size, relatively short follow-up, and incomplete data collection of each child's progress at every interval. The shortcomings in the design of the outcome studies were extensively used by critics of the implantation, claiming that most of the studies contain unspecified numbers of prelingually and postlingually deaf subjects; that individual data are rarely presented; that mean scores are often not representative due to the exceptional performance of some children; that investigators omit non-users from their series, thus artificially inflating children's performance; that many series have a selection bias by deliberately selecting only those children who can do particular tests; that the results obtained from small series are not generalizable; that no suitable control data have been used (Lane, 1995; Lane and Bahan, 1998). In addition, the formal 'laboratory' type tests that are used in the routine evaluation of implanted children may not reflect the child's everyday performance at home or school and assessments by parents and clinicians may differ widely (Vidas, Hassan and Parnes, 1992).

Data collected from Nottingham Paediatric Cochlear Implant programme includes all children except those described above who were explanted; it includes measures which capture the realities of everyday functioning such as Categories of Auditory Performance (CAP) and Speech Intelligibility Rating (SIR) alongside standardized measures such as the Edinburgh Articulation Test. The 'softer' measures such as CAP and SIR have had repeatability studies carried out on them and have been found to correlate with other measures which may be considered more objective. Measures of speech perception and production include those that can be carried out in young infants, based on video analysis and those which can be used with older children.

Speech perception

One study of open- and closed-set speech perception carried out over 5 years followed a consecutive group of prelingually deaf children after implantation. 83, 55, 32, 21 and 15 children reached the 1-, 2-, 3-, 4- and 5-year interval respectively. The study group was confined to prelingually deaf children aged between 2 and 7 years at the time of implantation. All were implanted with the same multi-channel cochlear implant system. No child was lost to follow-up and there were no exclusions from the study other than one child with auditory nerve aplasia. The Iowa Matrix Closed Set Sentence Test and Connected Discourse Tracking were used to assess closed and open set speech perception respectively without lip-reading. Children who could not do the tests were scored 0. The raw data for both tests and at all intervals were given in detail. The conclusion of the study was that prelingually deaf children who received cochlear implants before the age of 7 years developed significant closed-set speech perception abilities, as measured by the Iowa closed-set sentence test, in less than 3 years after implantation. Their ability to perform open-set tasks without lip-reading, as measured by Connected

Discourse Tracking, was limited in the first 2 years but showed significant improvement, not reaching a plateau, at the 4- and 5-year interval after implantation (Figure 9.2 and 9.3) (O'Donoghue et al, 1998).

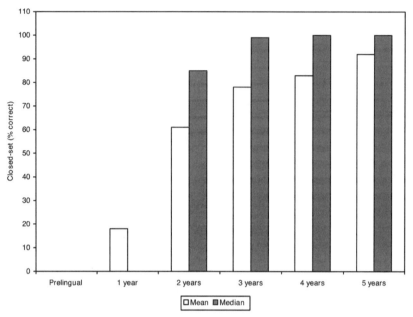

Figure 9.2 Assessing closed-set speech perception expressed as per cent correct on the IOWA Matrix Test (level A) before and up to 5 years after implantation.

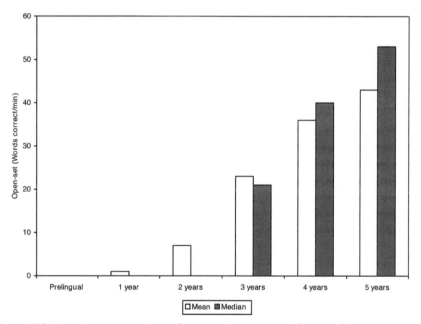

Figure 9.3 Assessing open-set speech perception expressed as words correct per minute in Connected Discourse Tracking before and up to 5 years after implantation.

Another study used the CAP to assess the progress of auditory perception in prelingually deaf children after implantation (Nikolopoulos, Archbold and O'Donoghue, 1999). CAP has been developed in Nottingham Paediatric Cochlear Implant Programme to reflect real life situations to which parents and professionals can readily relate and to bypass shortcomings of formal 'laboratory' type tests. (Archbold, Lutman and Marshall, 1995) It comprises an 8-point hierarchical scale of auditory perceptive ability, from no awareness of environmental sounds, through awareness and discrimination of speech sounds, to understanding conversation without lip-reading and the ability to use a telephone with a known speaker (Table 9.1). It is appropriate for use with young deaf children and can be used over an extended time frame without encountering floor and ceiling effects. CAP inter-observer reliability has been formally validated and high rate of agreement has been found between observers (Archbold, Lutman and Nikolopoulos, 1998).

In this study, a consecutive group of profoundly deaf children was followed up to 6 years after implantation (103, 77, 52, 30, 21 and 11 children reached the 1-, 2-, 3-, 4-, 5- and 6-year interval respectively). The study group was confined to prelingually deaf children aged between 2 and 8 years at the time of implantation. No child was lost to follow-up and there were no exclusions from the study. The results revealed that prelingually deaf children showed significant improvement in the auditory perception with implant experience. 82% of children who reached the 6-year interval could understand conversation without lip-reading. The respective percentage in the 3-year interval was 44%. None of the children could discriminate speech sounds before implantation (Table 9.1) (Nikolopoulos, Archbold and O'Donoghue, 1999).

Table 9.1 Categories of auditory performance in young prelingually deaf children (actual numbers at each interval)

	Category of performance	Pre	1Y	2Y	3Y	4Y	5Y	6Y
7	Use of telephone (known speaker)	0	0	5	6	5	7	3
6	Understand conversation (no lipreading)	0	3	13	17	16	8	6
5	Understand common phrases (no lipreading)	0	24	40	24	6	4	1
4	Discrimination of speech sounds	0	69	19	5	3	2	1
3	Identification of environmental sounds	5	6	0	0	0	0	0
2	Response to speech sounds (e.g. 'go')	4	1	0	0	0	0	0
1	Awareness of environmental sounds	14	0	0	0	0	0	0
0	No awareness of environmental sounds	110	0	0	0	0	0	0

Speech production and intelligibility

To assess speech intelligibility of implanted deaf children in real life situations, a 5-point hierarchical scale was also developed in Nottingham Paediatric Cochlear Implant Programme (Table 9.2) (Dyar, 1994; Allen, Nikolopoulos and O'Donoghue, 1998). This was also formally validated for inter-observer reliability and high rate of agreement between observers was established (Allen et al, 2001).

Table 9.2 Criteria used to categorize children using the speech intelligibility rating (SIR)

SIR criteria	
Connected speech is intelligible to all listeners. Child is understood easily in everyday contexts	Category 5
Connected speech is intelligible to a listener who has a little experience of a deaf person's speech	Category 4
Connected speech is intelligible to a listener who concentrates and lip-reads	Category 3
Connected speech is unintelligible. Intelligible speech is developing in single words when context and lipreading cues are available	Category 2
Connected speech is unintelligible. Pre-recognizable words in spoken language, primary mode of communication may be manual	Category 1

Profoundly deaf children were followed up for up to 5 years after implantation (84, 56, 32, 19, and 11 children reached the 1-, 2-, 3-, 4-, and 5-year interval respectively). The study group was confined to prelingually deaf children aged between 2 and 7 years at the time of implantation. The results revealed that after cochlear implantation the difference between the speech intelligibility ratings significantly increased each year for 4 years. For the first 2 years the median rating remained 'pre-recognizable words' or 'unintelligible speech'. It was not until the 3-year interval that the median intelligibility rating became category 3 (intelligible speech if someone concentrates and lip-reads). At the 4-year interval 85% of children had some intelligible connected speech. This improvement continued and at the 5-year interval, the median speech intelligibility was category 4 (intelligible speech to a listener with a little experience of deaf speech) and the mode was category 5 (intelligible speech to all listeners). The conclusion was that prelingually deaf children gradually developed intelligible speech that did not plateau 5 years after implantation (Figure 9.4) (Allen, Nikolopoulos and O'Donoghue, 1998).

Linguistic outcomes

Natural language acquisition is a complex process which is likely to be adversely affected by profound deafness from birth. Mellon (2000)

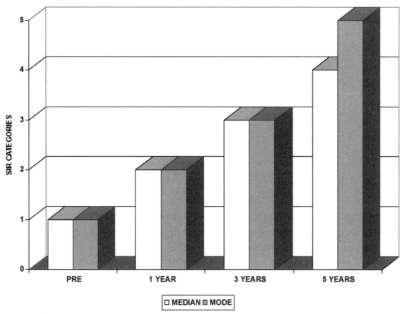

Figure 9.4 The median and mode of speech intelligibility rating (SIR) in prelingually deaf children after implantation.

provides a useful overview of the topic in relation to cochlear implantation. The main conclusions were:

- Multiple systems of skills related to language acquisition undergo development and this development is subject to a critical period (optimal time for refining the nervous system).
- Systems develop simultaneously rather than in series.
- Language acquisition depends on innate and experiental factors.
- The timing of first language acquisition affects linguistic competence.
- Specific processing requirements of the language acquired may determine cerebral organization for language.

The rate of language development in implanted profoundly deaf children has been found to exceed that expected from unimplanted profoundly deaf children (Tomblin et al, 1999; Svirsky et al, 2000) and the gap between chronological age and language age that normally widens over time in unimplanted deaf children remains constant after implantation (Miyamoto, Svirsky and Robbins, 1997).

The grammar development of spoken language was assessed in 38 profoundly deaf children implanted under the age of 4 years, using the test for reception of grammar (TROG), and was compared to that of age-matched hearing children (Nikolopoulos et al, in press). All children were implanted with the same multi-channel cochlear implant system. At the 5-year interval, 36% of implanted children performed at a level similar to (25–75 centile) or better (>75 centile) than the average hearing child of the same age. The respective percentage at the 3-year interval was 13% (Figure 9.5). Although the development of spoken language grammar in profoundly deaf children was found delayed in comparison to their hearing peers, it has been significantly enhanced by cochlear implantation. New advanced speech strategies and improvements in cochlear implant technology may allow further progress of deaf children in the development of spoken language.

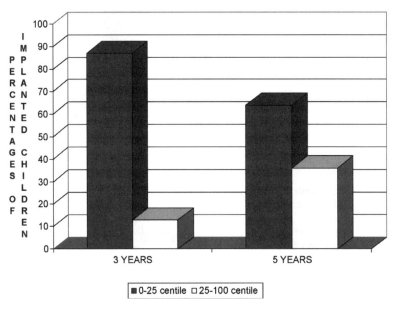

Figure 9.5 Performance of young implanted (<4 years old) children on the comprehension of grammar of spoken language (TROG results) in comparison to their hearing peers of the same age (centiles of hearing children).

Management decisions and cochlear implantation

Cochlear implantation has brought together the medical and educational worlds; has a medical intervention influenced management and educational decisions?

Communication approach

The two major decisions that parents make about the management of their child are how and where they should be educated. The choice of communication approach is made early in a child's life and may depend on many factors, including level of hearing loss. We explored the relationship between the approach to communication and measures of speech perception and production 3, 4 and 5 years after implantation (Archbold et al, 2000). The communication approach used by each child was classified by his or her Teacher of the Deaf at each interval, into one of two categories: oral communication and signed communication. Oral communication included only those children who used spoken language for communication entirely at both home and school; signed communication therefore includes a range of approaches, all of which use sign to some degree. At all intervals, those children who used oral communication significantly exceeded those who used signed communication on measures of speech perception and intelligibility ($p < 0.05$). However, when the oral group at 3 years after implantation were divided into those who were always oral and those who had used sign and changed to oral communication by 3 years after implantation, and their results compared, there was no significant difference between the two groups. It remains to be determined whether the children do well because they are using oral communication or whether they change to oral communication because they are doing well.

Educational placement

The last 20 years have seen an increasing trend towards the inclusion of all children in mainstream schools. Cochlear implantation, providing audition and access to spoken language to profoundly deaf children, could facilitate the inclusion of deaf children in mainstream education. Francis et al (1999) found that children with more than 2 years of implant experience were mainstreamed at twice the rate or more of age-matched children with profound hearing loss who did not have implants. Although they used age-matched groups, the sample size was small; there were 10 children with hearing aids and 10 children with more than 2 years of cochlear implant experience and all the children were in total communication settings, not reflecting the full range of educational provision. The Nottingham Cochlear Implant Programme examined the educational placements of 121 profoundly deaf children before cochlear implantation and 48 children who have reached the 2-year interval (Archbold et al, 1998). This study also examined the influence of age at implantation and duration of deafness on the placement of these children and compared the educational placements 2 years after surgery, of those implanted prior to schooling, and those implanted when already in a educational setting. Categories used were pre-school (P), school for the deaf (SFD), unit or resource base within a mainstream school (U) and full time mainstream provision (M). Age at implantation and duration of deafness were found to be significant predictors of placement 2 years after implantation. The duration of deafness of children in school for the deaf, or units, was double that of those in mainstream education. Fifty-three per cent of children who were in pre-school at the time of implantation, were found to be in mainstream schools 2 years after implantation. The respective percentage of children who were already in educational placements at the time of implantation was 6%. This difference was statistically significant.

The overall results indicated that children implanted early, before the educational decisions, were more likely to go to mainstream schools than the profoundly deaf children in the UK. However, the study compared young children with cochlear implants with the entire age-range (2–16 years) of children with hearing aids in the UK, and results were tentative.

A further study compared the educational placements of 42 profoundly deaf children with cochlear implants 3 years after implantation with the educational placements of 635 age-matched severely and 511 age-matched profoundly deaf children with hearing-aids, controlling for the effect of age (Archbold, Nikolopoulos et al, 2002). All 42 implanted children were implanted before beginning school in order to control for difficulties in changing educational placement. Three years after implantation, 38% (16 children) of the implanted children were found in mainstream schools, whereas 57% (24 children) were in a unit in a mainstream school, and 5% (2 children) were in schools for the deaf. Of the age-matched profoundly deaf children with hearing aids 12% (63 children) were found in mainstream schools, 55% (281 children) in a unit of a mainstream school, and 33% (167 children) in schools for the deaf. In the age-matched severely deaf children with hearing aids, 38% (239 children) were found in mainstream schools, whereas 51% (326 children) in a unit in a mainstream school, and 11% (70 children) in schools for the deaf (Figure 9.6).

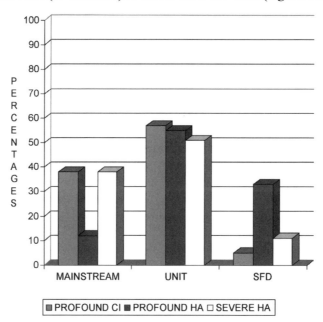

Figure 9.6 Distribution of educational placements among three age-matched groups of deaf children.

The statistical analysis revealed that there was a highly significant difference between the educational placement of profoundly deaf children with implants and those with hearing aids ($p < 0.00001$), whereas there was no statistical difference between profoundly deaf children with implants and severely deaf children with hearing aids. The conclusion was that profoundly deaf children, implanted before beginning school were attending mainstream schools 3 years after implantation in the same proportion as the severely deaf rather than profoundly deaf children of the same age with hearing aids. This conclusion has significant implications for the cost-effectiveness of paediatric cochlear implantation and for the future management of profoundly deaf children. Indeed, another study estimated significant savings in educational costs resulting from cochlear implantation enabling profoundly deaf children to function as severely deaf children in educational settings and that these savings contribute to cost-effectiveness (O'Neill et al, 2000).

Influences on outcomes

It is important to consider the factors which may influence progress. We have already referred to two: age at implantation and mode of communication. In order to explore these issues further, 40 prelingually deaf children were followed-up for 5 years with no selection or exclusions. The influence of five potential predictors (age at implantation, number of inserted electrodes, aetiology of deafness, mode of communication and socio-economic group) on speech perception was analysed. The speech perception assessment that was used was Connected Discourse Tracking where the child has to repeat a previously unknown story, phrase by phrase, without lip-reading, and the number of words per minute the child can repeat is scored. Clearly, the more the child is able to process the spoken language through hearing the faster the results on this test. Mean scores were 0, 27, 35 and 45 words per minute before implantation and at 3, 4 and 5 years after implantation respectively. Repeated measures analysis of variance revealed that children showed a statistically significant progress over time ($p = 0.001$), between all the intervals studied. Age at implantation and mode of communication at the interval studied were found to be significant determinants of the outcome (O'Donoghue, Nikolopoulos and Archbold, 2000). Number of inserted electrodes, aetiology of deafness (congenital or postmeningitic), and social class of parents were not found to have a significant correlation with the outcomes.

Parents' perspective: their views and expectations

Parental expectations relating to the success of cochlear implantation are considered so important that decisions about postponement, rejection, and selection of children for implantation have been based on these expectations (Kampfe et al, 1993). Moreover, parents should be considered as partners in the long education of implanted deaf children and their input is critical for children's progress. However, the literature is very limited in investigating their perspective. Kelsay and Tyler (1996) found that advantages and disadvantages expected by parents preoperatively were consistent with those reported by parents whose children had used their cochlear implant for 1–3 years. However, their results were considerably weakened by the relatively small number of subjects and the non-longitudinal character of the study, with different parents participating at the various intervals (only one parent participated at all intervals).

A longitudinal study was carried out in 43 parents of implanted children in order to assess their views before, and at 1, 2, and 3 years after implantation (Nikolopoulos et al, 2001). Three key domains were evaluated annually:

- communication with others
- listening to speech without lip-reading
- the development of speech and language.

The results revealed that pre-operative expectations were met or surpassed at each of the follow-up intervals. In the area of communication, 81% of parents expected a definite improvement pre-operatively, and 3 years after implantation 98% actually saw such an improvement. The respective percentages in the area of listening to speech were 35% and 88%, and for speech development 86% and (again) 86%. Speech development was the major area of concern at all intervals, illustrating the importance of the issue and the need for long-term studies in order to assess speech production that may need more than 3 years to develop (Figure 9.7).

In order to have a robust measure of parental views, the Nottingham programme has also developed and validated a special parental questionnaire, based on their open responses 3 years after implantation (Archbold, Lutman et al, 2002). This has been found to be robust and repeatable (O'Neill et al, submitted). Content analysis of the open questionnaires revealed the three most common constructs to be mentioned by parents: the positive changes in confidence (linked to communication) seen in their children, the need for continuing links with the implant centre, particularly for technical support, and the importance of

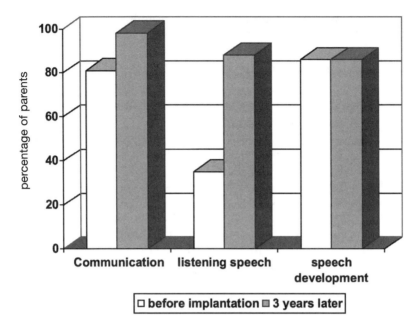

Figure 9.7 Percentages of parents expecting a definite improvement in their children in three key areas and the percentages of parents who actually note this improvement 3 years after implantation.

liaison between the educational service and the cochlear implant centre. The closed questionnaire has now been externally validated and will be used to explore the perceptions of larger numbers of parents in the long-term.

Long-term outcomes: educational attainments and employment opportunities

Although cochlear implantation has been available for 12 years, the long-term outcomes and possibilities are only just becoming apparent. The educational attainments of deaf children have long been the subject of study (Powers et al, 1998) and old studies such as that of Conrad (1979) are still quoted as showing the poor reading attainments of deaf children. It is important the attainments of children after implantation are carefully monitored, particularly for those implanted early. Does the early provision of useful hearing provide access to language acquisition in such a way as to make the attainment of age appropriate reading skills a reality for many profoundly deaf children? Unfortunately, the literature is extremely limited with regard to reading skills of implanted children. Moog and Geers (1999) studied 22 profoundly deaf children and found that the ratio of the reading age to the child's chronological age was 80% or above for 19 of the 22 children. These excellent results need to be confirmed by further prospective and longitudinal studies in the reading skills of implanted children. However, these encouraging indications urge us to continue to monitor this area, and those of ensuing further educational opportunities and employment.

Further areas of research

In recent years, early hearing detection and intervention programmes for identification of infants with hearing loss have become well established in many countries. In the UK, 20 areas have already started to implement a newborn hearing screening programme and all English health authorities will be participating by 2006. This will dramatically reduce the age of hearing loss detection and subsequent referral, when appropriate, to cochlear implant centres. Therefore, in the very near future, early cochlear implantation (at an age well under 2 years) will be an option for most children born profoundly deaf. We know that earlier is better; do we know that that earliest is best? (Gregory, 2001).

There is research and clinical data which indicate that the critical and sensitive period(s) for language development begin in the 6th month of fetal life and may be most susceptible to impairment during the first 2 years of life (Ruben and Schwartz, 1999). In addition to the possible existence of critical periods for language learning, there is a complementary argument supporting the importance of young age at implantation. The gap between chronological age and language age that normally widens over time in unimplanted deaf children seems to remain constant after implantation (Miyamoto, Svirsky and Robbins, 1997). In consequence, the earlier the implantation is performed, the smaller the gap between chronological and language age will be. Therefore, it is not surprising that young age at implantation has been found to be one of the most significant determinants of the later functional outcome (Fryauf-Bertschy et al, 1997; Cheng, Grant and Niparko, 1999; Nikolopoulos, O'Donoghue and Archbold, 1999; Nikolopoulos et al, 2000; O'Donoghue, Nikolopoulos and Archbold, 2000). Unfortunately in these studies the data are very limited with regard to children implanted younger than 2 years of age and therefore there is a compelling need for studies involving such children. However, preliminary evidence has demonstrated the feasibility of surgery with no significant complications and good early functional results (Waltzman and Cohen, 1998; Hehar et al, 2002).

Cochlear implantation in very young children will be a considerable challenge to teachers for the deaf and speech and language therapists, because most of the outcome measures are designed for much older children who have the communication skills to participate in the specific tasks. Therefore, there is a great need for development of methods to assess the early listening, communication and linguistic skills of these deaf children. Many of the outcome measures covered in the research described here are suitable for the very young. Nottingham Paediatric Cochlear Implant Programme is in the process of developing a package of measures appropriate for monitoring young deaf children with hearing aids or cochlear implants. The outcome measures included in this early assessment package will be language-independent, easy to administer and accessible to non-specialists, time-effective and useful over the short and long-term. They will enable those working with young deaf children to obtain a picture of the use of audition (whether by hearing aids or implants) in the development of spoken language. This information will enable management decisions such as whether to pursue the use of hearing aids or cochlear implants, which communication approach is the most appropriate and help identify the presence of other learning difficulties which may impinge on progress. Thus research and audit can influence practice and enable the support of the deaf child to be guided by facts rather than by rhetoric.

Chapter 10
Pilot study of a two-channel compression hearing aid with school age children

WENDY McCRACKEN

Relatively little research has focused on the use and potential benefits of new hearing aid technology for children. This study was designed to investigate the use of a two-channel aid, Multifocus, and to consider whether it is an acceptable management option for children. Previous trials had been encouraging but had been carried out on adult subjects. This trial included 25 school age children with each child acting as his or her own control to address the problem of multiple variables between subjects. The trial employed a simple crossover design between their own aids and the Multifocus aids. The child wore first one set of aids for a period of 12 weeks and then the other for 12 weeks. As Multifocus has no volume control, blind trials were impossible. The trial period was 12 weeks to allow for acclimatization effects (Gatehouse, 1993). Two sets of measures were used at the end of each trial period to allow comparisons of the children's performance with the two sets of aids. First, the THRIFT test of speech perception was used to test the aided ability of the children to perceive a variety of speech pattern contrasts. (THRIFT is the *Three Interval Forced choice Test* of speech pattern contrast perception; Boothroyd, 1995.) Tests were undertaken in both quiet and noise. Secondly, questionnaires completed by children's Teacher of the Deaf (ToD), parents and the children themselves were used to consider use of the hearing aids in a variety of listening situations. Finally, at the end of the trial, children and parents were asked to express a preference for one set of aids or the other. An informal post hoc questionnaire relating to the children's ongoing experience provided a window on to a currently unexplored area of the children's perceptions of hearing aid benefit.

Validation: assessing benefit of amplification

On-going validation of hearing aid benefit seeks to ensure that benefit predicted within a clinical setting is realized in the daily experience of the hearing aid user. Benefit may be measured through objective tests of speech perception and through self-report measures in a variety of listening situations. In addition benefit can be measured through reduction of disability as reported by significant others, for example: parents, spouses, teachers, peers, employers. In the case of deafened adults a number of measures have been developed to assess hearing aid benefit including:

- Profile of Hearing Aid Performance (Cox and Alexander, 1991)
- Abbreviated Profile of Hearing Aid Benefit (Cox and Alexander, 1995)
- Gothenburg Profile (Ringdahl et al., 1998).

Measures of benefit frequently focus either simply on audibility of the spoken word measured in a free field, or on using real ear measurements. Such measures are clearly important but are only a starting point.

Challenges

Assessments of the outcome of hearing aid fitting in children rarely look beyond the initial verification of fitting. Clinical reviews will often include a simple question to the primary carer and possibly the hearing aid user to establish whether there are any major problems that need to be taken into account. Hearing aid reviews are routine and follow set procedures, with little evidence that such reviews include consideration of individual hearing aid users, their lifestyle, their specific listening needs or the specific problems encountered.

Tests of speech perception

Tests of speech perception aim to provide an objective measure of how much more easily a hearing aid user can access speech with hearing aids than without them. There is a range of such tests. These vary from the relatively simple, where there is a lot of redundant information, for example a sentence test, to demanding tests where clues are minimized and the listener must rely solely on acoustic information perceived. In order to identify a suitable test of speech perception the final application of test results needs to be considered. Dillon and Ching (1995) provide a review of tests of speech perception including sentence, word and phoneme perception including the linguistic, phonemic and acoustic context of each test, the target group, response mode, ability tested and number of items per test.

Validation of paediatric hearing aid fitting

The effectiveness of the hearing aids in providing access to the auditory environment, in allowing children to hear themselves, family, friends, teachers, music and environmental sounds need to be assessed. The listening environment will vary from quiet to noisy, from being near to the sound source to being at a distance and from being acoustically friendly to acoustically hostile. Speech tests can be used with children to evaluate the effectiveness of hearing aids in the same way as they can for adults. In addition a range of subjective outcome measures can be used by children and their families. These include: Family Expectations Worksheet (Palmer and Mormer, 1999); Infant Toddler Meaningful Auditory Integration Scale (Zimmerman-Phillips, Osberger and Robbins, 1997); Abbreviated Profile of Hearing Aid Performance in Children (Kopun and Stelmachowicz, 1998).

Technological framework

The introduction of compression amplification in the 1970s, where the amount of gain varies according to the input level, offered considerable advantages to listeners – without the distortion associated with peak clipping (for a detailed summary readers are referred to Dillon, 2001). Research studies confirmed that listeners gained advantages from compression amplification (Hawkins and Naidoo, 1993). An advantage is that speech recognition for low level speech in quiet situations is improved with compression, especially for listeners with narrow dynamic ranges (Dillon, 1996). The potential benefits of compression amplification in noisy environments have been less evident in the research (Peterson, Feeney and Yantis, 1990; Moore et al, 1992; Dillon, 1996). Compression has been found to have a number of specific benefits for those with sensori-neural hearing loss: normalizing loudness, increasing comfort, controlling maximum output, reducing inter-syllabic intensity differences and controlling long-term variations (Dillon, 2001).

Listeners' preference for compression, the fact that background noise is predominantly low-frequency in composition and that high-frequency information is the area offering intelligibility, presented a challenge to researchers. Research began to focus on the possibility of splitting the speech signal into two bands and applying compression to each separately. There could be additional benefits for listeners, as sensori-neural hearing loss tends to vary across the frequency range, typically with a greater loss in the high frequencies, thus two-channel compression could take such a variation into consideration. In considering subjective reports of benefit and speech recognition in noise, some limited advantages were reported for adult users (Lawrence, Moore and Glasberg, 1983; Moore and Glasberg, 1986; Moore et al, 1992). Within the studies relating to two-channel non-linear compression, two studies demonstrated that speech recognition in noise was enhanced by the application of compression to the low-frequency band and linear amplification to the high-frequency band (Brunved, 1994; Williams, 1994). This finding is somewhat contradictory as it might be expected that more compression limiting would be required in the high-frequency channel. It is, however, suggested that linear amplification in the high-frequency channel coupled with non-linear amplification in the low-frequency channel is beneficial for speech perception because:

- compression reduces spectral contrasts that occur most importantly in the high-frequency band and that are important for speech perception
- in noisy situations the increased vocal effort of speakers gives increased high-frequency emphasis, and linear amplification allows this to be taken full advantage of
- it results in a near normal perception of the wearer's own voice, otherwise dominated by low frequencies at the hearing aid microphone (Bamford et al, 1999).

This approach had been tried with some success on adult hearing aid users (Olsen, 1992; Peterson, 1993; Biering-Sorensen et al, 1995) but only one study had been undertaken with children (Peterson, 1993). Although the results of this study were encouraging, it was based on only eight subjects.

The study undertaken here aimed to assess the potential benefit of this specific dual-channel aid in comparison with the children's own aids fitted optimally. It is, however, important to place such studies in context of our level of understanding. With respect to current advances in hearing aid technology, our ability to match these to the listening needs of those with sensori-neural hearing loss is restricted. Since our understanding of impaired cochlear function is limited (Moore, 1995), this limits our ability to take maximum advantage of the technology available and to adjust hearing aids to best meet the needs of the listener (Dillon, 1996).

Measuring speech perception

Speech tests can be used to determine the relative effectiveness of electro-acoustic characteristics of different hearing aids (Dillon and Ching, 1995). Speech tests may employ a range of test materials including toys, pictures, sentences, word lists and lists of nonsense words. In all cases, the stimulus is auditory and the objective is to assess the ability of the listener to access auditory cues. The response required, the time lapse, the quality of the test situation and the marking protocol will all affect the score obtained. The THRIFT measure (Boothroyd, 1995) was originally designed to test speech perception abilities of deaf children too young to undertake routine speech audiometry. THRIFT relies on a touch screen or mouse-controlled response. It employs nonsense words within an oddball paradigm, thus subjects are required to identify one signal that is different from two others: a forced choice test of speech pattern contrast perception. THRIFT contains nine subtests, each subtest containing twelve presentations that are defined by a phonologically contrastive dimension. As with all tests of speech perception, THRIFT seeks to measure audibility by providing an individual profile of access to phonologically significant speech pattern contrasts. This score provides a measure that is predictive for the development of sentence like speech perception performance. It also seeks to remain insensitive to current knowledge and skills.

Specific challenges within a paediatric study

Primary reports of benefit

The challenges presented to sensitive assessment of benefit in a paediatric trial are considerable. Research studies have tended to focus almost exclusively on adult subjects. These studies do not provide a basis from which it is possible to extrapolate potential benefits to children. Such studies most commonly use adults with acquired hearing loss. The cause of deafness, age of onset, educational experience, linguistic skills and social context of such hearing aid users is markedly different to that of children with permanent childhood deafness. The primary use of amplification for those with adult acquired hearing loss is to be a communication aid, supporting access to a known code, the spoken word, and use of spoken language. For prelingually deaf children, amplification is a way to access spoken language as one of the means to support the acquisition of that language. When sensitively fitted and appropriately managed, hearing aids offer the opportunity for some real advantages to be accrued by children with permanent deafness. It is however, only possible to ensure that full advantage of such benefits are achieved and that the hearing aid wearer is a full partner by actually measuring the benefit obtained.

Secondary reports of benefit

Fitting and verification within a clinical setting should be complemented by ongoing validation of the hearing aid fitting over time. This critical aspect of the amplification provision process is frequently overlooked. Validation is part of the recursive process, where the benefits and limitations of the amplification option are assessed over time in a variety of situations. The input from a variety of adults central to the child's experience and from the children themselves should be used to identify whether the goals of the hearing aid fitting process have been achieved. Such goals include audibility of the signal, clarity of the signal, comfort, and resistance to the interference of noise in the majority of daily situations for the individual child.

Listening environment

Personal amplification needs to offer maximum electro-acoustic flexibility if it is to meet the needs of a paediatric population. Speech itself is dynamic, fluctuating in respect of intensity and frequency. Children live and learn in noisy environments, both at home and at school. Children are demanding hearing aid users, actively involved in exploring their environment, in listening in halls, classrooms, the playground and on the street. The noise floor, reverberation time, spectral composition of noise and of speech, the vocal effort of the speaker and proximity of the hearing aid user to that speaker will all vary throughout the day. Background noise is known to be predominantly low frequency (Egan, 1988), this is particularly problematic for hearing aid users as speech intelligibility is carried predominantly by the less intense high frequencies. Environmental adaptations such as carpets and curtains to reduce background noise are useful to decrease reverberation, but also absorb high-frequency components more than low (Berg, 1997), thus reducing speech intelligibility.

Choice of speech perception measure

There are many tests of speech perception, but for the purpose of this study it was important to have a test that would maximally measure speech perception but minimally measure language skills, world knowledge and literacy skills. Additionally the measure should be easy to calibrate, to ensure that each subject received the same intensity of input, with the same spectral balance, presented at the same angle of azimuth. The response mode should require minimum motor, cognitive and linguistic skills and should not reflect the subject's phonological system, but engage the subject sufficiently to motivate completion of the test. This requirement precluded use of live voice presentation and of tests requiring verbal or written responses. It was important that the response mode did not require reading skills. A written response would be likely to favour older subjects and unreasonably disadvantage younger subjects. No single measure can appropriately evaluate speech perception because of the complex interactions that occur between the speech stimulus, context and knowledge and skills. In view of this a questionnaire was also employed to investigate perceived benefit

Study design

Full details of the study, test protocols and procedures are available in Bamford et al (1999). It was undertaken in collaboration with Sheffield Service for Hearing Impaired Children, the local health care trust and Oticon Ltd, and was designed to consider the efficacy of this novel approach to amplification with a group of school-age children. In conducting any trial that includes a paediatric population a number of challenges have to be addressed. Initially it was important to find an educational area that would be willing to take part in a field trial. Of necessity, such trials make extra demands on staff time, children's time and family time. The pressure of National Curriculum requirements and school timetabling need to be sensitively handled. Additionally, the eventual outcomes for the children were unknown and there is always a possibility that negative outcomes may ensue, such as: deterioration in speech perception, real or perceived; withdrawal from the trial, unwillingness to try out the usual aid if allotted the different aid first, or unwillingness on the part of the subject to complete the test materials. A paediatric field trial is further complicated by the relatively high incidence of middle ear effusion, unknown acclimatization effects and concerns over the ability of individual children to cooperate verbally with questionnaires. Furthermore, within the remit of this study, sufficient numbers of subjects had to be found with the appropriate audiological profile. This profile included that subjects should be established hearing-aid users, with no history of poor compliance, a flat or positive slope sensori-neural loss, with low-frequency thresholds between 25–80 dB HL and within the high-frequency band thresholds of 35–90 dB HL and with no conductive overlay.

Subjective measures of hearing aid benefit

An essential feature of this study was to ensure that the child and those closest to the child should report on their perceptions of benefit from a two-channel aid. As the child is the direct hearing aid user, it was important to ensure that provision was made to obtain the child's view of amplification options provided. Somewhat surprisingly, this is a relatively novel approach. Standard practice focuses on specific fitting protocols, and on real ear measures of gain. The individual child's view on a specific amplification option may be sought in a clinical review, but little effort has been put into ensuring children's opinions and experiences have been accounted for and valued.

Changing listening needs of a paediatric population

The individual lifestyles of children make considerable demands on amplification. The rapid changes characterizing the first year of life in respect of proximity to speaker, angle of azimuth and direction of microphones as infants move from prone to sitting, crawling and walking have been considered in the literature. There is little evidence of clinicians taking into account the lifestyles of primary school or secondary school children, despite the fact that technology offers increasing electro-acoustic flexibility. The individual lifestyle preferences of children, their preferred listening situations, the importance of audibility balanced against cosmetic preferences, control preferences, ability to hear and monitor own voice, the feeling of 'connectedness' with the immediate environment are some of the important variables that affect acceptance of personal amplification.

Perceived benefit in a paediatric population

This study sought to ensure that each individual child's opinion was sought and incorporated into measurements of benefit as far as possible. A self-completion questionnaire was developed that included questions relating to eight typical listening situations, based on work carried out at the MRC Institute of Hearing Research (Grimshaw, 1996). The aim was to ensure that parents, teachers and children all completed similar questionnaires, appropriate rewording was used and a categorical approach using pictograms included for the children. In addition children completed the questionnaire in an interview setting to ensure ease of access and to promote full responses. This important but subjective measure was complemented by the use of an objective measure of speech perception.

Challenges in self-report approaches

In seeking to measure subjective benefit from amplification, the use of self-report scales presents some specific challenges. The situations chosen should have real-world face value. It is important to represent situations that the hearing-aid user is likely to encounter on a regular basis, thus it is important to consider both place and qualities of listening environment. Such situations would naturally include poor listening situations with competing background noise and a long reverberation time. Additionally, children are required to listen to teachers in classrooms as well as in the playground, to parents in quiet and in noise and to use amplification to gain information about the world around them, for personal safety and for enjoyment. Each of these facets can be incorporated within a listening benefit scale but comparisons across a group are challenging. The degree of background noise, its spectral composition, the reverberation time of a particular listening environment, the distance from a specific speaker may vary considerably. Situations that may be typically important for one age group, for example. listening to a CD, may not typify the experience of a subject with permanent childhood deafness, whereas access to a television programme may be important. The quality of the sound from a specific television, the distance at which the subject sits, the use of direct input and FM system, the volume control setting are all important factors. In addition, the acoustics of the room in which the television is placed will all be important factors that should ideally be taken into account for the individual listener.

Test protocols

Decisions regarding the test protocols and instrumentation were aimed at ensuring consistency and rigour and at being appropriate for the range of subjects within the hearing aid trial. In order to ensure that the introduction of a new hearing aid did not prejudice subject responses, great care was taken with the type of language used to describe the two-channel aid. The clinician had to ensure that loaded vocabulary suggesting that 'different' was in any way 'better' was avoided. It was impossible to run a blind trial, as the aid chosen for this study, (Multifocus) has no external volume control. The range of subjects also made comparisons across the group problematic: for this reason, each subject acted as his/her own control. At the end of the trial children and parents were able to choose to keep the preferred hearing aids (own or Multifocus). Hearing aid provision within the UK is provided through the National Health Service and is free at the point of delivery. This service includes regular clinical reviews and updates of technology as appropriate. It was concluded that financial concerns would therefore not bias the trial. All the personal hearing aids fitted before the trial were refitted according to a standardized paediatric protocol (Seewald, 1992). Desired Sensation Level (DSL) is a paediatric fitting protocol that provides target sensation levels for the long-term average speech spectrum as a function of threshold at each frequency. These measurements in turn provide real ear gain targets for the individual. If direct uncomfortable loudness level measures are not available, this procedure also provides targets for real ear maximum output values based on thresholds. Additionally, measurements of middle ear function were important, as this would preclude subjects experiencing conductive overlay from the trial period or would allow it to be taken into account during the trial.

Test conditions

The choice of test conditions raised a number of important questions:

- At what signal-to-noise ratio (S/N) should the aids be tested?
- Should each subject be tested at the same signal-to-noise ratio, or

should a 50% response rate be calculated for each subject to ensure that no one was working at ceiling level for the test?
- What type of noise should be employed for the listening-in-noise test situation?
- How adverse should the S/N ratio be?

The poor acoustics in schools are well documented (Berg, 1997), as is the importance of a positive S/N ratio, an ideal of +24 dB suggested by Markides (1986), for children with sensori-neural hearing loss. Against this, it was important to ensure that subjects were able to complete THRIFT in a clinical setting within the time allotted and before fatigue or habituation concluded the test. It was also important to reflect what was actually realistically achievable in a classroom or home situation. Test conditions with a S/N ratio of +5 and 0 were agreed. In order to ensure that the background noise equally affected all speech sounds, classroom babble shaped to the long term average speech spectrum was used. The decision was taken to test all subjects at the same intensities. To this end, presentation of speech stimuli was controlled by PC soundcard via two speakers at a distance of 60 cm and 45° angle at each side of the touch screen. Presentation was at 60 dB(A) measured at the subject's head. For the presentation in noise, a second set of loudspeakers were mounted on top of the signal loudspeakers. In this test situation the S/N ratio at the subject's head was 0 dB.

Acclimatization issues

Timing of the study was an important consideration. It is standard clinical practice within the UK for a hearing aid review to include an audiogram, middle ear measurements, electro-acoustic checks of the hearing aids and real ear measurements. New personal aids may be fitted through the same process and verification of the fitting, assured by employing a paediatric fitting protocol and real ear measures of gain. For a paediatric population, there is little evidence of acclimatization effects being considered. Studies by Gatehouse (1993) and others suggest that for deafened adults, an acclimatization period of 12 weeks is necessary before benefit can be sensitively considered. In the case of prelingually deaf children, there is no reason to suppose that a shorter time-frame is appropriate for such measures. It could be argued that an even longer adjustment period may be needed when new technology is prescribed, and this may well be the case with fully digital technology. As research probes these questions it is important that the user of the technology is put centre stage within this process, that those fitting personal amplification listen to what children have to tell us. Within this research study the crossover took place at 12 weeks after measures of benefit were obtained.

Study design

The study was designed to compare the appropriateness of a two-channel aid compared to the subject's 'best fit' OAs. The two-channel aid used was Oticon Multifocus (MF) where wide dynamic range compression is applied to the low-frequency channel and linear amplification with peak clipping is applied to the high-frequency channel. Peak clipping is applied at relatively low levels for linear instruments, ANSI high frequency average of 109 dB SPL and 119 dB SPL for middle and high-powered instruments respectively used within this study. In the low-frequency channel, a knee-point lower than 50 dB SPL means that compression circuitry is always active. This setup allows the low-frequency components typical of background noise to be compressed along with the low-frequency but relatively intense components of speech. In contrast, high-frequency components of speech and the spectral contrasts important for speech recognition are given maximum amplification. MF has its own fitting strategy that takes into account the configuration of the individual subject's audiogram, and the dynamic range of hearing in the low and high frequency bands. The design of the trial involved one centre and employed a simple crossover design. A total of 25 subjects entered the study, 7 male and 18 female, with an age range of 6.2 to 14.9 years with mean pure tone average hearing levels in the range 54.7–59.5 dB HL (averaged thresholds). It was important to ensure that OA and MF were matched for size and colour to avoid these issues clouding decisions regarding preference. Aids were fitted according to the appropriate protocol, fine-tuned within a week with the help of a hearing-aid diary completed by the child and family. It was important to monitor middle ear status to identify and treat episodes of otitis media with effusion. End-point measures were employed at the crossover visit and at the end of trial. Despite concerns relating to the time needed to complete tests in quiet and noise, all subjects were able to remain on track and complete the tasks required.

It was interesting to note that although the MF fitting protocol is based on adult field trials, there was evidence of MF fittings closely approximating the fitting targets of the DSL protocol. Results demonstrate no advantage of OA or MF aid when testing was conducted in quiet conditions. For both types of aid, there was a predictable advantage in vowel contrasts over consonant contrasts. Tests in noise resulted in lower scores for both types of aid. In noise there was, however, a clear advantage in favour of MF aid over OA. Statistical tests were employed to assess any carryover or order effects. In all cases no evidence of such effects were identified.

Questionnaire responses

Composite scores were calculated for each questionnaire, with a total score for each respondent in the range 24–12. In all three groups (child, parent and teacher) the score was higher for MF than OA, reflecting perceived benefit. ANOVA demonstrated the treatment differences in all three groups were statistically significant. At the end of the trial children and parents were asked to choose which set of aids they wanted to retain: 76% of the children expressed a preference for MF over OA whereas 86% of parents preferred MF to OA. These preferences were significant and were attributed by the respondents to clarity of speech, performance in noise and volume control.

Summary of findings

In assessing benefit, both THRIFT and the questionnaire scores demonstrated significant effects in favour of the two-channel aid. In addition, the final preference questionnaire completed at the end of the study indicated a clear preference by both the hearing-aid wearers and their parents for the two-channel aid. The questionnaires to teachers were interesting in that they gave markedly lower scores relating to perceived benefit than either of the other groups. It may have been that teachers were more critical in their appraisal, had lower expectations, or that children and parents had raised expectations. The non-random allocation of subjects to treatment groups could have led to bias or sampling error, although post hoc examination of the cases failed to identify any significant differences.

Children as active research participants

A post-hoc phone survey with those ToDs involved in the study was undertaken to get a feel for the continuing experience and level of satisfaction expressed by the children who had been involved in the study. There was no attempt to talk to the children themselves or to undertake any statistical analysis of results. Rather it was an opportunity for advantages and disadvantages that had come apparent to be identified. Of those teachers who could be contacted the following comments were made:

> For the first time she can wear her aids at dinnertime. This is a real plus because there is so much going on at lunch-time in the hall.

> He keeps them switched on when swapping lessons. The corridors can be very noisy and he always turned the others off.

> The twins both report that they do not feel so tired at the end of the day. Maybe they don't have to put so much effort into listening.

> The real problem is she won't wear the radio aid now, she really thinks she can do without it. I am going to wait and see how she gets on. I remain to be convinced.

I am not sure it's anything to do with the new aids. He used to have headaches all the time and spend lots of time in the unit at playtimes. He says the new aids don't give him headaches . . . but who knows.

These comments suggest there may be a range of potential benefits that are important to individual hearing aid wearers, but at present we have no appropriate measures that consider these. Comfort, reduction of stress in noisy situations, reduction in cognitive effort when listening in noise, ability to tolerate a wide range of signal inputs are all important aspects of hearing aid acceptance. More importantly such reports underline the ability of children with permanent childhood deafness to report benefit and preferences.

Children are clearly able to actively participate in formal tests of benefit but additionally, as users of the amplification, have important information to share with service providers regarding their lifestyle, specific listening needs and preferences. Both acclimatization effects and the importance of the ongoing validation process in hearing aid fitting should not be underestimated. The hearing-aid user, whether adult or child, should take a central role in the process of ensuring appropriate amplification is fitted and modified over time to meet changing needs. Children are the end-users of amplification and therefore have the potential to add considerably to our understanding of benefit. Simple application of an essentially adult-based model of hearing aid benefit is likely to underestimate the importance of a child's perspective. The challenge for researchers is to find new ways of unlocking this evidence. By listening to what children have to tell us about their experience of amplification, new perspectives can be brought to bear and our understanding of the process can be broadened and enriched.

Chapter 11
Investigating text support for deaf students

RACHEL O'NEILL AND AILSA LAIDLER

Educational context

This chapter explores one aspect of support for deaf students in further education: text support. The research was funded by the Viscount Nuffield Auxiliary Fund and allowed City College Manchester to employ a researcher for a year.

Further education for deaf students in the United Kingdom has always been strongly vocational, but in the past 30 years, vocational education has moved out of residential school trade departments and into further education (FE) colleges (McLoughlin, 1987). When deaf students started to enter FE for day release courses in the 1970s (Green and Nickerson, 1992), colleges started to recruit the first communication support workers (CSWs). Over the past decade another specialist support role has emerged: notetakers for deaf students. The project investigated three different types of text support for deaf students in FE and compared their effectiveness. The project team wanted to discover which deaf students would benefit from each system, and the practical constraints that may appear when these systems were introduced into an FE setting.

Research context and literature review

There has been very little research in the field of post-16 education in the UK. Deaf education has been no exception to this British research trend, so much of the evidence base comes from the United States. The research summarized here includes discussion of interpreter as well as text support in the mainstream classroom because these are alternative, and sometimes complementary, forms of communication support in post-secondary education.

187

Stuckless, Stinson and colleagues in the National Technical Institute for the Deaf (NTID) with Rochester Institute of Technology (RIT) in New York State, USA have pioneered research which explores students' perceptions of text support in the classroom. First they examined the use of stenography, an American phonetic transcription system used by court reporters for verbatim records (Stuckless, 1983). Then they conducted surveys of deaf students' views on the system (Stinson et al, 1988). They found that for students who came from mainstreamed schools, the Real Time Graphic Display was more intelligible than an interpreter and more helpful than handwritten notes. This was the first time real time text had been used to test student comprehension, and the researchers realized that the dysfluencies in speech, for example false starts, incomplete sentences, ungrammatical constructions and repetition, could lead to lower comprehension scores. They concluded that one method of communication support does not suit all students, because students from residential schools who had better-developed American Sign Language (ASL) preferred an interpreter in class.

In England, researchers at Bristol University (Wood and Kyle, 1989) trialled a computer notetaking system at Bristol university called Hi-Linc. They used a BBC computer which allowed some technical terms to be pre-stored; their operators were mainly secretaries rather than trained notetakers. The researchers examined speed, accuracy and intelligibility of text and looked at the number of idea units that the operators were able to convey, as an attempt to compare hardware and operators. The term 'idea unit' was not defined clearly in their research, but was based on the core meaning of clause elements. This research noted that operators who had experience of notetaking with deaf students were better at summarizing ideas than operators who had a secretarial background.

In the mid-1990s, Gallaudet University hosted a conference to examine the implications of inclusion, or the least restrictive environment, as American legislation refers to it. Deaf and hearing presenters challenged the view that the mainstream class was the least restrictive environment for deaf learners. Stinson and Lang (1994) discussed group learning, which is obviously important for all students and particularly difficult for deaf students in mainstream settings. They also discussed the poor quality of many educational interpreters, and reported that deaf students did not always remember information relayed via an interpreter.

Researchers in Mayfield, Kentucky (Youdelman and Messerly, 1996) used an Apple Mac computer linked to a TV display in mainstream classes with five profoundly deaf participants. The subjects usually used lip-reading and reading handwritten notes. These students found they were able to join in the classroom discussion much better than with handwritten notes. The researchers also outlined the qualifications needed for electronic notetakers which have been adopted in the UK by the exam board CACDP (the Council for the Advancement of

Communication with Deaf People): good summarizing skills, a high level of English skill, a word-processing speed of 60 words per minute or above, an understanding of deaf education issues and impartiality.

At NTID Stinson et al (1996) investigated deaf students' views about different communication methods in the class. Deaf students who used speech felt more confident at communication with hearing peers. There was considerable variation between deaf students in the same class about how comfortable they felt with hearing peers and tutors. The discussion raised the issues about the difficulties deaf students face if they work with an interpreter in a mainstream class, and how their psychological feeling of separation can grow. They concluded that deaf awareness from the usual class tutor at the start of the teaching year may help deaf and hearing students communicate more easily and allow everyone to work better with the interpreter.

Rawlinson (1998) raises issues of the effects of introducing real-time captioning into mainstream classes. She discusses the Americans with Disabilities Act (ADA) of 1990 and the case of a tutor who objected to transcripts being given to deaf students in a class because hearing students do not get them. She reports the interpretation of the ADA that a transcript should be made available to hearing students too if they pay for the copying. The tutor does not have the right to forbid real-time captioning in class.

Foster, Long and Snell (1999) examine the views of deaf and hearing students at RIT, which is predominantly a higher education institute. They found that there was no great difference in the views of deaf and hearing students about classroom communication, but deaf students were more concerned about the pace of instruction and they did not feel so much that they were part of the institution. The teaching staff reported that they made few modifications for deaf students and saw this as the role of the support staff. The article suggests some practical guidelines for preparing tutors to work in a more inclusive way.

Over the past decade the team at NTID in Rochester has developed a new software package called C-Print, where speed typists are trained to use a system of abbreviations in order to increase their output speed. The operator types on one laptop and the output is conveyed to another, which the student reads. Elliot et al (2001) administered questionnaires to 36 college students and interviewed 22. Students rated the comprehension with C-Print to be higher than their understanding of the interpreter and they preferred the C-Print printout to handwritten notes. Students who were relatively proficient in literacy and speechreading preferred C-Print to an interpreter. NTID and RIT have 1200 deaf students, and many come from mainstream schools where they have used speech rather than ASL.

Much of this research is based in higher education settings; FE is characterized by more participative teaching and learning styles. The fact that there is more interaction in the FE classroom means that it is even more important for deaf students to have live access to discussion with peers and tutors. It will also be important for deaf students who use British Sign Language (BSL) to have a clear way to intervene in class. One way is through an interpreter or CSW, and a less satisfactory way is through the student writing or word-processing questions to the support worker.

Research questions

Research undertaken at City College Manchester explored three different systems of text support for deaf students:

Manual notetaking

The deaf students sit next to the notetakers, reading everything that happens by looking at their notepads. The notetakers pass the sheet to the students as soon as it is finished. Manual notetakers are trained with a 21-hour course and a deaf awareness certificate. They are often graduates with good English and summarizing skills and neat, quick handwriting. In the classroom they write down everything that they hear, including comments and asides from the students, noises off and interruptions. The speed of speech in the classroom can reach 200 words per minute, but a good notetaker can only write about 50 words per minute, so this form of text support necessarily summarizes.

Electronic notetaking

With this form of text support the deaf student reads a summary of what is happening in class on a laptop. Electronic notetakers are usually recruited in the same way as manual notetakers, but they have a word-processing speed of at least 60 words per minute. They work with two laptop computers, which are joined with a serial cable so the deaf student can read the proceedings easily without peering. The software used for this project was C-Note, a shareware programme from Queen's University, Canada (see Appendix). C-Note is two-way software, so that as well as students reading the proceedings, they can also type questions which the operator reads out.

Towards the end of the project the college was able to trial Speedtext and Stereotype, two more effective programs developed by the RNID and Sheffield Hallam University respectively. Stereotype is one-way software, because it is designed to be used in lectures where the deaf students can ask questions using their own voice, or via an interpreter. Speedtext is two-way software: the deaf student can type questions back to the operator who then voices the question to the class. Both systems also have a dictionary which allows the operator to store abbreviations of technical terms. There is a marked difference in the price of these software products: Stereotype is much cheaper than Speedtext.

Palantype

Palantype is a phonetics-based keying system, different from qwerty keyboards. The operator has lengthy training to reach speeds of over 180 words per minute. Several keys are pressed for each phoneme or consonant cluster. Most Palantype operators work in courts, and because of their contracts are not free to work in educational settings. Some Palantypists have become interested in educational work with deaf students and taken a deaf awareness certificate. The Palantype equipment is also expensive and has to be programmed with technical subject words before a class. The printout from a Palantype session can be bulky, because it is a verbatim record. The transcript contains all the usual dysfluencies of spoken language, which can make it difficult for a weak reader to understand.

Aims

The aims of the research project were:

- to examine deaf students' perceptions of different forms of text support in education
- to investigate the practical considerations about providing Palantype or qwerty text transcription, including e-mail or disk transfer of files soon after class
- to produce a report which will inform deaf educators and trainers of text support workers.

Tutors and CSWs at the college recognized the need for more specialism of roles within the team. The team wanted to find a cost effective way of training well-qualified support staff who would give deaf students good access to the course content as well as the life of the classroom. Many deaf students entering FE have stronger skills in English than in BSL, although a CSW using stage 2 or 3 BSL is often the only support staff available. (For details of UK educational levels see the next section.) One solution to improving the quality of communication support is to train CSWs to interpreter level (i.e. National Vocational Qualification in BSL at university level, or Level 4) because BSL is the first choice communication method for many adult deaf students. Another solution is to train effective text support workers to use English, and this may suit students who arrive at college with reasonable English literacy but weak BSL skills.

The project team consisted of a worker (the second-named author of this chapter) and a project management team that included a deaf student representative, a deaf tutor, two advisors based in universities and a tutor of deaf students from the college who supervised the project (the first-named author).

Methodology and participants

The students taking part in the research were studying on a typical range of FE courses, from Entry level to Level 3.

- **Entry level** on the National Framework is at levels 1–3 of the UK schools National Curriculum, approximately equivalent to Grades 1–4 in the US education system.
- **Level 1** is at the National Curriculum Levels 4–5, or Grades 5–9 in the US system.
- **Level 2** courses in the UK include the A–C grades of the General Certificate in Secondary Education (GCSE), or work which is usually expected of a school student at 16. In the US this would be work at 11th grade.
- **Level 3** courses include the UK Advanced level, between 12th grade and an Associate Degree in US terms.
- **Level 4** is university level work, which is the main focus of the previous American research, is at level 4 on this framework. (BSA, 2001:4).

Table 11.1 Student participants and their courses

Student	Age	Full- or part-time	Course	Level
A	43	PT	History of Art Open College Network	3
B	19	FT	General National Vocational Qualification, Advanced Business	3
C	28	PT	City and Guilds 7307 Teacher training	3
D	25	PT	National Vocational Qualification Horticulture	2
E	17	FT	Certificate in Childcare	1
F	19	FT	Foundation Studies	E

The three text systems were demonstrated to students at college open days and a group of six students volunteered to try each system in one of their classes for at least three weeks each. The Edinburgh Reading Test (1977) was administered to four of the six students.

The grant from Nuffield allowed the college to buy Palantype equipment and laptop computers.

The British examination board CACDP now has a qualification in electronic notetaking, but this was not available in 1999 (CACDP, 2000), so the electronic notetakers on the project were trained in the support team for deaf students at the college. All the electronic notetakers had

Table 11.2 Language and reading profiles of student participants

Student	Preferred or stronger language	Reading age if tested	Usual in-class support	Degree of deafness
A	Spoken English	Has a Higher National Diploma	2 CSWs co-working, interpreting from BSL to English	Severe from age 1
B	Sign supported English	12;2	1 CSW interpreting and sometimes a manual notetaker too	Profound from birth, fitted with a cochlear implant a year before
C	British sign language	Has a degree	2 CSWs co-working interpreting from BSL /English and a manual notetaker	Profound from birth
D	Spoken English	10;6	Radio aid and manual notetaker	Severe from birth
E	British sign language	9	CSW who uses BSL/ English interpreting	Profound from birth
F	Spoken English	7;6	CSW who uses clear speech, some SSE and notetaking	Severe from birth

an induction to their role, but they were the least trained at the time of the trials. The manual notetakers taking part in the project had the CACDP Level 2 Certificate in Note-taking for Deaf People qualification and deaf awareness training, and the Palantypists had the CACDP Deaf awareness qualification.

Data collection

- Student perception questionnaire of each type of support and the usefulness of the notes.
- Tutor perception of the support worker in class and the accuracy of the notes.
- Usual support worker's observation of communication.
- Tape recording and verbatim transcript of one session in each mode.
- Comprehension questions after each session: 10 questions, the first 5 without the notes to assess their in-class understanding.
- Student views ranking each system and comparison with usual support.

Methodological/ethical issues

Not all the data collected was analysed. The aim originally was to compare the structure and detail of the notes with the transcript of the tape recording to look for the number of omissions or errors with each system, and if possible, the structuring of ideas in lectures. This process proved too time-consuming. The comprehension questions at the end of the third session with each system were not always a good indication of comprehension of the particular session, because some of the questions could be answered by using background subject knowledge. The main data source for this project was the perception questionnaires completed by the participants.

In the City College Manchester trials there were some ethical dilemmas about withdrawing the usual support from deaf students. One student (E) withdrew from the project after trying only Palantype because it was so much worse than her usual CSW support. A second student (C) decided not to try the manual notetaking as she had found the other two systems gave her less access than her usual communication support, which was interpreting.

Results

Manual notetaking

Students C and E did not try this type of support because they felt they would not get enough information in class. Student B used the notes, but asked for the CSW to continue to support her in class because she could not get enough information through just a notetaker. This meant that only the three severely deaf students felt comfortable about working with a manual notetaker.

It was interesting to see the points at which student B turned to the CSW for clarification, unwilling to rely solely on manual notes:

- to check meanings of new terms in the handouts
- to find out the reason for background noise she could hear through her cochlear implant
- to join in the discussion with a voiceover from the CSW
- towards the end of the session because she was tired.

Students and tutors rated the handwritten notes very highly: as easy or very easy to read and understand. They were regarded as useful by all students for reference after the class, for revision and for writing assignments. However, manual notetaking could not provide information quickly enough for those students who relied on notes to find out what was happening in the class.

Student comments included:

- It was a bit boring and a bit slow. (A)
- There is not enough information (B)
- I tended to read the notes when the notetaker had finished the page, so there was a big delay. (A)

- I have very little access when the only form of support is that of a notetaker (C)

The students scored well in the comprehension questions designed to test the information they had gained from the notes during the class. This is probably because the notetaker includes all essential information, omitting a lot of the miscellaneous detail. So although the students do receive all the key information, they don't receive it at the same time as their hearing classmates, and they don't get the 'feel' of the class. They also often miss out on the conversations between students, which are important for friendships with hearing peers.

Only student D rated manual notetaking as his favourite form of in-class support. He made good use of residual hearing and used lip-reading well in class too, so he did not rely just on the notes to find out what was happening in the classroom.

Electronic notetaking

Student E withdrew from the project before trying this method of communication support. The training background of the three electronic notetakers used for the project varied. One was an electronic notetaker in higher education while the other two had only recently been trained and had only worked in this role for a number of weeks. This had an impact on the students' experience of the support.

All the notes were rated highly by students for their inclusion of useful information, but student evaluations of the layout and clarity of the notes varied. The more experienced notetaker was able to produce notes with a clearer layout in live mode, e.g. use of paragraphing, topic headings, sub-headings, clear sentence structure, etc. These features made student comments more favourable.

The electronic notetaker's ability to use the hardware and software effectively also affected their speed. Less experienced operators did not have enough time to note non-essential information. This often resulted in conversations between peers, which are valued by deaf students, not being recorded. Because of these omissions, all the students reported that their usual form of support provided them with more information.

Students also reported that it was 'quite hard' to concentrate on the screen all the way through a class, and two noted that it was physically tiring. Watching the screen also meant that students missed out on visual information from the class, as well as sense of human contact with classmates.

An example from student C's class showed that reference was not always clear in the notes. The tutor sometimes referred to 'you', which the electronic notetaker recorded but it was not clear who it meant. Similarly when the tutor pointed to something and said 'Make a note of this', it was not clear what the student had to do from the notes. These issues of layout and reference need to be addressed thoroughly in the training of electronic notetakers.

Some tutors found the noise of the keyboard distracting in early sessions with an electronic notetaker, but a few weeks later reported that they had adjusted to it quite well.

Student comments included:

- A good text summarizer can produce more information than a note-taker, and includes all the main points. There's no waste or junk as there is with Palantype.(A)
- The structure of the notes was not clear enough. My questions were joined on to the tutor's lecture. (B)
- I felt bored and tired looking at the screen instead of my usual support, which is an interpreter. (C)
- It gave me the chance to make my own notes after class using the disc. (D)

Palantype

All students tried this method of text support. The responses to this system varied considerably, and the features which some students regarded as strengths were regarded as weaknesses by others.

Palantypists aim to produce a verbatim record of speech, so the text output has a number of features which are different from the text produced by electronic notetakers:

- the number of words in the text is far greater:
- there are dysfluencies which match speech exactly
- nonsense words sometimes appear because the operator has not got the word stored in the computer's dictionary

Three students, A, B and C, identified the quantity of text as an advantage: they could have access to the same information as their hearing peers, including comments, asides and jokes from their classmates.

The Palantypist needs information before the class to input technical terms and proper names which may arise. No Palantypist can achieve 100% accuracy, so the student has to deal with spelling errors, non-words and miskeyed words. For students who do not have enough subject knowledge or knowledge of the English language, decoding these errors can be impossible. The same sorts of errors can be seen on live subtitling of news programmes.

Student perceptions of how easy Palantype was to use varied from 'a bit difficult' to 'quite easy'. Students felt they grasped 'about half' to 'most' of the classes with Palantype. Most students found it hard to concentrate for the duration of the class.

Some tutors were alarmed that every word that was said would be recorded. They evaluated the printouts after each class, and some said they felt uncomfortable knowing that the full transcript was going out of their class.

Comments from the students included:

- Occasionally I could not work out mis-spelt words, names or terminology, which made understanding difficult. I was not sure what the tutor was talking about. (A)
- It is very high English. I do understand what most of the words mean, but I can't understand it. (E)
- It gave me new vocabulary to learn from. (B)
- I knew what conversations students were having. I knew who was saying what and I knew exactly what was going on. (B)

The final notes were rated highly by those students who were confident in English, because of the amount of information included, but generally the Palantype notes were poorly rated for clarity and structure.

Discussion

Selecting students for text support

The research project allowed the deaf student support team to have a clearer idea of which students were most likely to benefit from text support.

Two students, A and B, who had previously received signed communication support in class, preferred electronic notetaking after the project because it provided a model of English language usage. They could see how to use technical vocabulary, and they felt they were not always getting this technical vocabulary via the BSL used by the CSW. This could be because the CSW did not have the necessary level of BSL vocabulary, or because the students preferred to see English because their assignments were going to be written in English.

It was noticeable that individual ratings of each system did not always correspond to an independent analysis of the notes. For example, student B rated the paragraphing in the Palantype notes very highly, when there was in fact very little paragraphing in the notes. Those students who had negative experiences in oral educational settings may have been negatively disposed towards text support even before they tried it, and so believed that it was difficult to understand.

Student F, who had the weakest reading skills of the students taking part in the study, did not find any type of text support particularly useful. She has some learning difficulties in addition to her deafness. She liked being able to refer to manual notes after practical classes, but the other two systems produced too much text for her to read.

Factors which the project team regard as good indicators of success with electronic notetaking or Palantype were that the deaf student should have:

- a reading level above 12 years (or success with Key Skills Communication Level 1 tests)
- a positive attitude towards English
- confidence in their own reading skills

These last two factors could perhaps be quantified by using an attitude survey such as the one developed at NTID in Rochester, NY (Stuckless, 1983).

Selecting trainee manual and electronic notetakers

The selection of trainee notetakers for the course leading to the British exam board CACDP's qualification Note-taking for Deaf People is very important and can have a great influence on the quality of the support workers. The following selection criteria apply to both manual and electronic notetakers:

- Before starting their training notetakers should have a good level of education, preferably a degree; high-level English language skills, for example Key Skills Communication Level 3 (see Appendix), good summarizing skills; clear, neat handwriting if they are going to be manual notetakers; a word-processing speed of at least 60 words per minute for electronic notetakers.
- Graduates are much more likely to have the necessary academic, spelling and summarizing skills.

Working with manual notetakers in FE

As a result of this project the deaf student support team decided to use manual notetakers less for live reference in class. The team recommends that these factors should determine the choice of a manual notetaker to work with a deaf student:

- the deaf student is hard of hearing or deafened, rather than deaf from a young age
- the student can use residual hearing or is an excellent lip-reader
- the notes are needed for backup, not for live reference in class.

Manual notetakers need some tidy-up time at the end of a class session, but the aim is that the student has the notes on the same day.

Working with electronic notetakers in FE

The current CACDP Note-taking for Deaf People qualification stipulates that electronic notetakers should pass a basic deaf awareness certificate before they study for an adapted version of the manual notetaking course. The CACDP Electronic Note-taking course focuses on the specific features of hardware and software that operators will use. As a result of this project, the deaf student support team recommends in addition that electronic notetakers need training in language modification to suit the reading levels of particular deaf students, including an understanding of the varieties of English which they may see deaf students typing. They should have CACDP BSL stage 2 so they can communicate with a wider range of deaf students. They need health and safety awareness training to ensure safety in class and to prevent repetitive strain injury. They need a greater educational awareness of the needs of deaf students, for example by completing the course run by the British exam board Edexcel: the Professional Development Award in Communication Support Work for Deaf Students.

As a result of this project, the deaf student support team at City College Manchester was able to draw up a job description for electronic notetakers, a code of practice for them and guidelines for class tutors for working with an electronic notetaker (see Appendix).

Electronic notetakers can improve the readability of the notes after class, and this usually adds 10 minutes to a one-hour class. An advantage of these notes is that they can be easily e-mailed to the students.

The deaf student support team at the college experimented with using electronic notetakers in other situations while the research project was running. The college has several courses for deaf students which are taught in BSL. These classes previously had a manual notetaker who translated from BSL to handwritten notes. At the end of the class the notes are copied and given to all students as a summary of the proceedings. Two members of staff in the deaf student support team had electronic notetaking skills as well as BSL skills at National Vocational Qualification level 3. They now provide electronic notetaking support for groups of deaf students on training courses taught in BSL. The printouts are rated more highly by students than manual notes because they are much easier to read. There is not currently a specific qualification to accredit these support skills

Working with Palantypists in FE

The project needed to book Palantypists as part of the research, but it emerged that it is very difficult to contract them for part-time work in education. As stated earlier, court contracts often prevent them from taking on other work. The rates of pay for Palantypists are currently similar to those of registered sign language interpreters.

A Palantypist needs time before class to set up a subject dictionary. This time becomes less as the course progresses. They also need tidy-up time after class to make the notes more readable and to produce the printout. The notes can also be e-mailed to students.

Although there is currently a national shortage of Palantypists, this may not always be the case. If better training were available, including training in deaf awareness and BSL, Palantype would be the preferred method of communication in class for some deaf students. In Sweden stenographers are trained to work in deaf communication roles and work in pairs on a rota basis, as sign language interpreters do. Stenography works on the same principles as Palantype. If there were professional training for Palantypists to work in deaf education in the UK, there would be some demand for them.

In a few years time, however, speech recognition software may well have improved so much that it will be able to record speech from several speakers in a classroom discussion in text form. Some students will want this level of detail and be prepared to put up with the dysfluencies of speech for the advantages of having a complete record (for more about automatic speech recognition, see Appendix).

Training needed for students in text support

Deaf students entering FE need time to see and try all the text support systems available, just as they need time to learn to work with a CSW or interpreter. If the student does not have good keyboard skills, going on a word-processing course would be helpful, as most text support workers are not proficient enough at BSL to be able to provide an accurate voice-over of the deaf student's questions or comments.

Practical considerations

There were some practical outcomes arising from observing text support in classes:

- Equipment has to be positioned near to an electric socket. On one occasion a student had to sit apart from other students to be nearer a power supply, even though there was an extension cable. Trailing wires had to be taped to the floor, and this took extra time for the operator to set up.
- Notetakers should try to position the student's screen so that it is directly facing the tutor or main speaker with a clear view to the OHP, flip chart or other visual media. Be aware of glare or reflections on the screen.
- Appropriate desks and chairs should be available to text support workers. Notetaking is a physically and mentally tiring task, for both

manual and electronic notetakers. An adjustable typing chair with good back support is very important.

- A lightweight, stable trolley is useful for moving laptop and Palantype equipment. Notetakers have to move heavy equipment between classes and sites on a regular basis.
- Security is an important issue both for storage and moving the equipment. A lockable cupboard in a locked room is needed. Staff are vulnerable when carrying expensive equipment, particularly between college sites.
- Electronic notetakers need to be confident at file management and printing, and know their software and hardware well.
- Students who use BSL rather than speech must have training in keyboard skills so that they can make contributions via the keyboard. This training will increase the confidence that students have in the system. Two-way software was essential for these students.
- Some practical courses, such as drama, are not easy to provide text support for. Students are usually embarrassed by the prospect of having live notes projected with a data projector. The electronic notetaker also has to be very confident to be prepared for all the class to see their live notes on screen.

The evolving role of the CSW

The research project led the deaf student support team to believe that more training is needed for all text support workers, so that they become a specialist form of CSW. The CACDP notetaker training does not give enough knowledge of the language learning background of deaf students, so trainee notetakers should also join the Edexcel Professional Development Award in Communication Support Work with Deaf Students. Stage 2 CACDP BSL is one of the entry requirements for the Edexcel course, so it may take some years before electronic notetakers have the BSL skills necessary to start training as a CSW.

The CSW is a type of professional in deaf education found in the UK but not in other countries. CSWs are trained to use a wide range of communication methods and to work in the classroom with deaf, hard of hearing and deafened students. They pass as much information as possible between tutor and students using whatever mode the deaf student prefers. This can include interpreting between BSL and English, moving from English to Sign Supported English, using notetaking, lipspeaking or deaf-blind communication methods. CSWs also modify written language into plain English at a level the student can read, and they often provide informal deaf awareness to the college lecturer and hearing peer group. (FE Guidelines, RNID, 2001)

The British exam board Edexcel offers a qualification called the Professional Development Award in Communication Support Work for

Deaf Students which provides knowledge of deaf students' educational experiences. CACDP, which examines BSL and other communication skills used by CSWs, has recently published a national code of practice and guidelines for employers to ensure higher standards (CACDP, 2001).

A national picture of undertrained CSWs and tutors of deaf students

In 2000 the National Association for Tertiary Education for Deaf People (NATED) conducted a survey of all FE colleges and sixth-form colleges that found 2818 deaf students in a survey with a response rate of 68% (O'Neill et al, 2002).

The NATED 2000 survey shows that 266 FE and sixth-form colleges support deaf students, with the average number of deaf students in each college being low: 1–9 students. The survey paints a worrying picture of poorly-qualified CSWs: only 31% of CSWs held the Edexcel certificate and only 27% had CACDP stage 3 BSL or above. Furthermore, specialist tutor support was not the norm; there were only 120 qualified tutors of deaf students working in 77 colleges. This leaves 71% of the colleges which support deaf students without a qualified tutor to assess their learning and communication needs. The 2000 survey did not ask specifically about the skills and training of notetakers and electronic notetakers; however, there are currently very few trained electronic notetakers in the UK.

In practice, it is often pragmatic considerations that determine who will support the deaf student. There is a shortage of BSL/English interpreters in the UK and educational interpreting is not a high-status specialism as it is in countries such as Sweden and Denmark. British interpreters rarely work in FE because working conditions are poor: it is rare, for example to find co-working, and colleges are reluctant to pay interpreter rates when a CSW with stage 2 BSL will work for half the pay. Learning and Skills Councils, which fund FE in England and Wales, need to be better informed about deaf students' need for registered interpreters who are working at National Vocational Qualification level 4. As interpreters can find better-paid work in community settings, courts or theatres, CSWs are left trying to interpret when they are usually not trained in this work. Recently there has been some criticism of the role of the CSW, because one person cannot communicate effectively in such a wide variety of situations, and because most CSWs do not have interpreter training (Harrington, 2001).

One approach to the national picture of an undertrained workforce is for colleges to employ both bilingual and monolingual CSWs. A bilingual CSW should be trained to interpreter level, and monolingual CSWs such as electronic notetakers or lipspeakers, would work mainly with English. Both groups would benefit from the training in educational support work and knowledge of deaf students' learning needs provided by the current Edexcel CSW course.

Initial assessment on entry to college

Initial assessment by a qualified tutor of deaf students working in partnership with a deaf BSL tutor or assessor is crucial for determining the student's needs. The National Association for Tertiary Education for Deaf People (NATED) has recently updated its assessment pack (2002) that includes an assessment of the deaf student's literacy skills, spoken language skills and BSL receptive and productive skills. The assessing team and the student working together decide on the type of communication support that the college will provide. The decision to choose text support or interpreting support is a complex one, and the student needs to be fully involved in the discussion about which method suits them best.

Conclusion and outcomes

The main outcome of this project was that the team re-evaluated manual notetaking and decided that electronic notetaking was generally more useful to deaf students in FE settings. For deaf students who use fluent BSL, text support is not a satisfactory alternative to a fully trained CSW or an educational interpreter. Many other deaf students, even some who use BSL, may be more oriented towards English and may prefer an electronic notetaker.

Electronic notetakers should be well trained with a thorough awareness of language modification for deaf learners, academically proficient and deaf aware. It is not a cheap or quick alternative to train electronic notetakers; these support staff need to have the same breadth of training as other CSWs. As one student in the project commented,

> With all the three text systems I tried, there's a difference between a good support worker and a not so good one. (A)

No one type of communication support will suit all deaf students and support teams need to have a range of trained staff to contract, depending on the individual deaf student's needs.

Acknowledgements

This research was made possible by an award from the Viscount Nuffield Auxiliary Fund. The authors would like to acknowledge participation in the project of the following: Fauzia Ullah, deaf student representative;

Vera Pickens, Tutor for Deaf Students; Mike Wald of Southampton University and Clare Gallaway of Manchester University, both project advisors.

Appendix: website resources and software

C-Print in Further Education, from the Rochester Institute of Technology in the USA: *http://www.rit.edu/~easi/itd/itdv01n2/cuddihy.html*

Current developments in Automatic Speech Recognition and deaf education: *http://netac.rit.edu/publication/asr.html*

Code of Practice for Electronic Notetakers from City College Manchester is available from Rachel O'Neill: *roneill@ccm.ac.uk*

Key Skills – used in Further Education to assess progress with communication, literacy and IT: *http://www.qca.org.uk/nq/ks/com_app_it2.asp*

Speedtext is available from the RNID, 19–23 Featherstone Street, London EC1Y 8SL. Contact Kerryn Krige: *kerryn.krige@rnid.org.uk*

Stereotype is available from Paddy Turner, Disability Support Manager, Sheffield Hallam University, Student Services Centre, Owen Building, City Campus, Pond Street, Sheffield S1 1WB: *pturner@shu.ac.uk*

Chapter 12
BSL/English interpreting in higher education: is access to the university curriculum a reality for deaf students?

NOEL TRAYNOR AND FRANK HARRINGTON

Over the past nine years, since the University of Central Lancashire (UCLAN) established its Deaf Studies programme, not only has the interest in Deaf Studies as a subject increased, but the university has also begun to develop a Deaf culture of its own. It has attracted Deaf and hard of hearing students on to a large number of different courses in a wide variety of departments and disciplines. From a small beginning in the early 1990s, the University now has a population of more than 60 deaf students, including 40 Deaf British Sign Language (BSL) users; it also has five Deaf lecturers and researchers whose first or preferred language is BSL.

In this chapter, we use the convention, as adopted by Woodward (1972), of using Deaf (with a capital D) to refer to BSL users who regard themselves as part of a cultural and linguistic minority; deaf (with a lower-case d) refers to students who do not use sign language. Where both groups are discussed, D/deaf is used.

With the steady and continuing increase in the number of D/deaf students at UCLAN, the university identified issues relating to access to the higher education system that had not previously been addressed. This led to the proposal of a second strand to an existing project, funded by the Higher Education Funding Council for England (HEFCE), which had been examining staff training, continuing professional development and students with disabilities; this second strand was to focus on the communication needs of Deaf students using sign language interpreters in the classroom, and to evaluate the effectiveness of interpreted classroom interaction.

Background

Perhaps the first noteworthy development in provision for deaf and disabled students in higher education occurred in 1948, when services for disabled students were established at the University of Illinois, USA. Anti-discrimination legislation over the past 35 years provided more of a real stimulus for change in the USA (Lane, Hoffmeister and Bahan, 1996); in European countries, however, there appeared to have been a conspicuous lack of interest in deaf and disabled students. In the UK, much attention was given to widening participation from under-represented groups, with the major focus being on women and people from minority ethnic communities.

Changes began to occur in the early 1990s, when the financial support available to full-time students with disabilities was increased considerably. In 1990 the Royal National Institute for Deaf people (RNID) commissioned research into access for D/deaf students in higher education (Daniels and Corlett, 1990); this work established that the existing service was not appropriate, and highlighted the need for improvement. The research recommended strongly that all higher education establishments should have an equal opportunities policy, and should also have a designated member of staff responsible for ensuring that the needs of D/deaf students were met. It further recommended that national organizations for D/deaf people should campaign to ensure that adequate government funds are made available to meet these needs.

The Further and Higher Education Act (HMSO, 1992) introduced single funding bodies for each national system of higher education institutions. In the same year, the Privy Council consented to the change of name from Lancashire Polytechnic to 'The University of Central Lancashire', and UCLAN became one of several new universities offering widening participation to previously excluded groups. With the establishment of Deaf Studies as a component of its combined honours degree in 1993, UCLAN set the stage for an influx of D/deaf students.

After the 1992 Act, the initial guidelines from the government required the funding councils to 'have regard' for the needs of students with disabilities. The four countries of the UK each adopted different strategies, although all four allocated additional funding to institutions to promote the development of policy and provision. Further advances followed the recommendations made by the Dearing Committee in 1996. In addition, the Disability Discrimination Act (HMSO, 1995) will, by the end of 2002, also have a direct impact on education provision for disabled students, and should help to ensure that the momentum continues into the twenty-first century.

What has happened in the USA and the UK is echoed to varying degrees in other countries. The result is that there are now more disabled students in higher education. Of these, many are D/deaf, and systematic campaigns in the UK for the official recognition of BSL as the UK's fourth indigenous language have helped to raise the profile of sign language users. After the 1992 Act, the new funding body responsible for universities, HEFCE, set up a working party with the necessary funding to highlight a variety of needs, in particular the needs of disabled students. One of these needs was acknowledged as being for sign language interpreters for Deaf BSL users, and it was on this that our research at UCLAN was to focus.

Opening the classroom door

Although a number of the HEFCE funded projects in 1993–94 and 1994–95 had focused on issues relating to Deaf students, much of their focus was on responding to the practical questions raised by the need to provide and fund access to institutions of higher education. These projects had concentrated on ways of establishing the students' support needs, finding personnel to provide this support, ensuring that the funds were available to pay for it, and establishing strategies for raising the awareness and improving the communication skills of staff who would be working with these students (HEFCE, 1996).

Other projects had concentrated on issues of physical access, and improvements were brought about by the provision of technical support for deaf students. Laptop PCs were acquired for students to borrow, as were text-phones and audiological equipment such as loops for hearing aid users. During the period from 1993 to 1994, 87 projects gained HEFCE funding; of these, only 28 focused solely on the needs of D/deaf students and deafness. Little actual research was done, as most of the projects were devoted to the provision of equipment and disability- or deaf-awareness training for staff. very few universities set up sign language interpreter booking systems, or provided Communication Support Workers (CSWs); only two projects established interpreter posts. Most of the projects appeared to concentrate their energies and funding on their own staff, increasing awareness and their ability to cope with widening participation in the form of disabled and D/deaf students.

In the early 1990s Disabled Student's Allowance (DSA) was relatively low, and was mainly available for technical and medical support. The 'non-medical helpers' component was small, and most often related to care and supervision costs. The increase in Deaf students meant that more high-calibre sign language interpreters were needed, and the average DSA fell far short of being able to pay for this: Members of the Register of BSL/English Interpreters (MRSLI) are expensive, and Trainee (TI) and Junior Trainee (JTI) Interpreters, although less expensive and less highly qualified, still cost far more per hour than care workers. By 1998 this shortfall was recognized, and the level of DSA for non-medical helpers tripled, thereby enabling more Deaf students to employ better-quality interpreters for their lectures and coursework. The result was that by the time of the project, many of the lectures in UCLAN had Deaf students in attendance with interpreters; at the same time, the increase in numbers of Deaf lecturers within the Deaf Studies programme meant that interpreters were also working to ensure access for hearing students.

The proposed second strand of this project would now provide a first opportunity for the project team to go beyond the more basic access issues. It would open the classroom door and investigate in more detail whether or not the support, once provided and funded, was actually effective. In doing this, the project team were not simply looking at the practices of individual interpreters, or identifying errors in the way they worked or the way they manipulated language. Rather, the project was looking at the entire classroom environment where there was interaction between an interpreter, a lecturer and Deaf and hearing students, with the aim of evaluating the overall success of communication within the process of education in which they were all participants and stakeholders.

Among the project objectives was the intention to take what was learned and use it to improve the situation for each of these groups of stakeholders; to improve access to the curriculum and the learning experience for Deaf students, to improve the training, skills, expertise and working practices of interpreters working in higher education, and to raise awareness and understanding of the communication differences necessary for lecturing staff to meet the needs of a Deaf student in their classroom. This last objective had a particular impact on the first strand of this project, that of widening participation, and is one of the pivotal points that brought the two strands of the project together.

The Project Officer team comprised one Deaf and one hearing researcher, the latter an MRSLI with a high level of expertise and experience in organizing and training sign language interpreters. Both were concerned to observe the level of communication support within the classroom, and were keen to discover the nature of support in other institutions as well as UCLAN. In the early stages of widening participation, little real funding had been available for interpreter support; consequently, in some cases it had been necessary to employ untrained and relatively inexperienced CSWs, many of whom are not trained in the use of BSL beyond the CACDP Stage 2 qualification.

The Deaf Project Officer (Sign Language) focused on the perspective of Deaf students using the interpreting service, and on the effect of being included in a lecture where the lecturer, perhaps, had little or no experience of Deaf students. His work and observations fed directly into the provision of awareness training for UCLAN staff within the first strand of the project. The hearing Project Officer (Interpreting) concentrated more on the practices of the interpreters who were observed; the impact they had on the learning environment, as well as the impact that the learning environment had on their ability to function effectively. He also explored the implications of these for sign language interpreter training and improvement of the service.

Research methodology

Review of relevant literature

In addition to the available information relating to the background to the project, much of which has been referred to above, it was important, in particular in relation to the second strand of the project, that the project team have a good understanding of previous work that has been done on sign language interpreting and interpreting in educational settings.

As has already been mentioned, earlier studies in the UK had focused mainly on the need to provide interpreters in higher education settings, and on the financial and other implications of achieving this. On the whole, however, the question of whether or not the services provided were appropriate or effective in giving students access to the curriculum had not yet been addressed.

In other countries, particularly in the USA, some significant research had been carried out in relation to the effectiveness of educational interpreting in primary and secondary settings (K-12), (see Winston, 1994, 1997). Even here, however, there was not a large amount of research or data relating directly to the effectiveness of interpretation in post-compulsory education, although that which did exist proved to be an important starting point for the project team (Johnson, 1992; Roy, 1993; Sanderson, 1997).

In looking at the university classroom setting as a place of learning for Deaf students, the team quite quickly became aware of how different an environment this is from the primary or secondary education settings in which deaf children are taught.

In school, students are supported by their classroom support worker, teacher aide or educational interpreter, whose roles, aside from communication, can be many and varied (Green and Nickerson, 1992:179–192). The students may spend much of their time being taught or supported on an individual basis, and, if they are not in a specialist school for the deaf, they may be with other deaf students in a partially hearing unit (PHU) for as much time as they are in class with their hearing peers (see Hopwood, this volume). It is also to be expected that their teachers will either have specific qualifications for working with deaf children, or will have received some training before having a deaf child placed in their class. It is clear that the school environment in which a deaf student is placed is, to a large extent, designed by those responsible, in an attempt to meet both the real needs and the perceived needs of that individual.

In a university setting the student's situation is quite different. In the UK, it is unlikely that the majority of university lecturers will have undergone any specialist training in disability or deaf awareness (Hurst, 1993). Lecturers expect to function in a situation where they share a common language with the students, and when they find an individual Deaf student in their classroom, supported by an interpreter and notetaker, it is our experience that many of them assume that they need make no other adjustments to the way in which they deliver their lectures.

The services that universities are able to provide for the support of students also vary widely in both scope and quality from one institution to another. Deaf students should, theoretically, have the opportunity to attend any university in the country, and to study any subject or discipline, but in practice this choice is often limited by the ability or willingness of institutions to provide the services necessary to meet the student's individual support needs (Barnes, 1996).

In terms of the actual interpreting support that students might require, various studies have been carried out (Kluwin, 1985; Winston, 1989; Mertens, 1991), which suggest that it is important to match the students' language needs in order to give them the maximum opportunity to learn and comprehend.

Collection of information

Information was collected nationally from interpreters who work in HE and from Deaf people who have received interpreter support while studying in HE. This information was collected mainly by questionnaires which were sent out in August 1997. The data from the returned questionnaires helped to build an overall picture of the level and success of both past and current provision for Deaf students in HE. This data was evaluated and formed an important part of the content of a several papers and presentations about the project.

In particular, it confirmed what the project team already suspected, that few of the best or most qualified interpreters regularly accept any educational interpreting assignments, and as a result most of these assignments are undertaken by people who have not undergone interpreter training or whose skills are less advanced. The implications of this were that students have a limited choice of interpreters to work with them, with those who are available having varied degrees of skill and ability. Finding an interpreter whose language skills match the needs of the student is difficult.

In addition to this the survey also highlighted the fact that there is no guarantee that individual interpreters have attended university themselves, or that they are knowledgeable in the subject areas for which they may be expected to interpret. In fact it had been suggested by the Council for the Advancement of Communication with Deaf People (CACDP), which is the examination and assessment board for interpreters in England, Wales and Northern Ireland, that as few as 5% of people interpreting in educational settings in Britain at the time the project was carried out possessed appropriate language skills and a graduate-level qualification. Such a lack of knowledge on the part of educational interpreters, either of the environment in which they are working or the subject they are interpreting, combined with lower language skills, would be bound to have an impact on the student's ability to learn (Harrington, 2001).

The general shortage of interpreters in the UK means that many deaf students are accessing higher education through the services of people who may not be trained interpreters, and who may not themselves have personal experience of studying at that level (Harrington, 2001).

Questionnaires sent to Deaf ex-students were also a valuable source of information. They gave exceptional insight into the experiences of Deaf students, and raised issues about the booking and funding of interpreting services, and about the appropriateness of individual interpreters in meeting the needs of particular students.

One point in particular that was highlighted was the possibility that Deaf students themselves may have come to university from an environment in which they had been supported throughout by a classroom support worker, and as a consequence, may not have had a clear understanding of how to work independently with an interpreter or notetaker. Combined with the observations made earlier regarding the qualification and experience levels of some interpreters, this will naturally have implications for the effectiveness with which interaction and learning will be accessed in the interpreted classroom.

In addition to the questionnaires, the project officers successfully applied to the operators of the MAILBASE electronic mail system in Newcastle University to establish a discussion list for BSL/English interpreters and those teaching and researching Deafness and interpreting. From May 1998 the Project Officer (Interpreting) coordinated this list, providing a forum for greater discussion between interpreters, Deaf people, national and regional deaf organizations and interpreter trainers from around the country. It proved to be a valuable source for further information about interpreters' and Deaf peoples' experiences of higher education and other related settings. Membership of this discussion list is now more than 120, and it continues to be a useful forum for the discussion of interpreting and educational issues.

Meetings with stakeholders

An early objective was for the Project Officers to meet the people who were to be stakeholders in the project (students, interpreters and lecturers), to discover their current experiences of interpreted lectures and to ascertain what outcomes they expected or wanted from the project.

Meeting the students was quite easy, especially at the start of the academic year, but it was more difficult to arrange a time to meet the interpreters, as most are self-employed, and not available to attend meetings. Consequently, the Project Officers had to contact them individually, initially by letter, and then in one-to-one conversation.

Contact with the lecturers was delayed for two reasons. First, until the students had been given fixed timetables it was not known which staff members would be teaching them. The university's own Specialized Learning Resources Unit (SLRU) needed timetables to arrange interpreters, and until these were settled nothing could be done. Second, the Project Officers had to wait until they knew which of the contacted interpreters were willing to be involved in the project before they knew which lecturers they could approach. The Project Officers again had to meet these individually, having first contacted them by letter, as, like the interpreters, few were willing or able to attend a meeting.

Persuading lecturers and interpreters to allow the project team to film them in action was no easy task; some interpreters perhaps would feel threatened by the presence of video cameras, while lecturers might regard us as intruders. Much individual discussion and reassurance was needed before we gained agreement from all the parties involved, and these initial meetings were an essential part of the project.

Video-recording and observational data collection

Observation and data collection were the key activities within the project, giving the Project Officers the primary data on which they could base their observations and analysis. Between November 1997 and February 1998 they observed and filmed 32 hours of interpreted lectures, collecting evidence involving 15 different lecturers across 8 subject areas, including Education Studies, Deaf Studies, Social Work, Counselling, 3D Design, Business Management, Social Studies and Computing.

In these settings, the Project Officers observed 11 individual Deaf students working with 9 different interpreters. The qualifications of the observed interpreters were as follows:

- 4 were Members of the Register of BSL/English Interpreters
- 3 were registered as Trainee Sign Language Interpreters

- 2 had not received any formal interpreter training, but had certificates in sign communication skills.

Two VHS video cameras were used to gather this evidence and, in line with the objectives mentioned above, the Project Officers filmed and observed not only the interpreter, but also the lecturer, the students, both Deaf and hearing, and the classroom environment.

Where possible, the Project Officers all also interviewed participants, to establish:

- how they felt about the session that had been video recorded and observed
- whether they felt everyone in the situation had been afforded equal access to the information which was being given
- what, if anything, they would wish to change about that situation.

The Project Officer (Interpreting), a first-language user of English, interviewed the Hearing people, and the Project Officer (Sign Language), a first-language BSL user, interviewed Deaf people. This ensured that everyone had the opportunity to comment in their first or preferred language. As both project officers continued to analyse the collected data, they asked individuals to view the tapes with them and offer further comments.

Project findings and developments

The findings of the project enabled the teaching staff, Deaf students and interpreters involved to put into practice what was learned.

Teaching staff

The main activity carried out by the Project Manager and the Project Officer (Sign Language) in relation to the first strand of the project, was raising awareness for university staff. They used findings from analysis of videotaped data during the delivery of these sessions, which influenced the information given to university staff regarding their use of interpreters in teaching situations. The videotape analysis identified a number of points that related specifically to the practices of teaching staff, and which might allow them to work more effectively with interpreters and Deaf students. These included:

- their use of other media in the classroom – overhead projectors (OHPs), televisions, videos, etc.
- their general awareness of the task and role of the interpreter, as well as of the Deaf student's needs

- environmental issues relating to the layout of teaching rooms, positioning of interpreter/Deaf students, etc.
- the need for them to prepare notes and materials (including video transcripts, etc.) in advance.

Suggestions for improved practice

On the basis of the project team's evaluation of the videotaped evidence, suggestions were made for changes in lecturers' style and delivery to accommodate the needs of interpreters and Deaf students. It was recommended that notes, OHP slides, transcripts of TV programmes and videos, etc., should be made available to interpreters and Deaf students before the session. Lectures and materials should be planned in advance so that these might be made available to interpreters in good time. It was suggested that OHP slides and other media should be left where they can be seen for long enough to enable Deaf students to look at them without missing what is being communicated by the interpreter. A pointer can be used to highlight a particular part of an OHP slide while talking about it; a book or other paper can be held up so that it can be seen while it is being talked about. Where possible, videotapes should be used with on-screen signing or subtitles; there should be regular pauses at appropriate points in presentations to enable interpreters and Deaf students to catch up with each topic, and ask questions if necessary. Participants should be positioned in such a way that nothing, including the teacher, can impair the sight lines and the communication process.

Where possible, rules should be introduced into the classroom so that overlapping talk does not impede the interpreter's ability to function effectively.

Deaf students

Both project officers were involved in the promotion of good practice for new and returning students regarding their working with interpreters. This happened in two ways:

- formally, as part of enrolment week at the beginning of semester 1 and advice week in semester 2
- informally, in conversations and discussions with individual students

Again, issues identified from the analysis of the videotapes included:

- the need for students to be clear about the role of the interpreter and of the teacher in the classroom
- the need for students to be more assertive in using the interpreter (stopping the interpreter for clarification, ensuring that they themselves have equal participation in and access to discussions and debates, etc.)

- the need to develop an appropriate and mutually useful working relationship with the interpreter, and how to move towards this.

Interpreters

Both project officers were involved in the interpreter training courses that the university offered, at both graduate and postgraduate level. In designing the curriculum for these courses, outcomes of the project led to the development of new modules on interpreting in public service and educational settings. The findings of the project influenced and informed the development of these modules. In particular, the Project Officer (Interpreting) was involved in the delivery of these courses in regional centres around the country from September 1998 and was, in addition, a member of the teaching team for existing interpreting related modules on the undergraduate programme within Deaf Studies. The Project Officer (Sign Language), as well as being involved with the Project Manager in teaching Disability and Deaf Awareness within the university, also organized and taught separate Deaf Awareness sessions as part of the university's undergraduate programme. He was also responsible for running BSL classes specifically designed to improve the communication skills of members of university staff. It is possible to see the positive influence and effect of the project in these activities, which had an impact on the university environment.

The analysis of videotaped data identified a number of issues for interpreters, some of which were outside of their control, but all of which had an effect on their ability to function effectively in the classroom. These included:

Preparation/subject knowledge

Preparation was highlighted above as something that could be improved by greater awareness on the part of lecturers of the needs of other participants in their classroom. It is one of the major factors which hinder an interpreter's ability to do as good a job as they might. One cannot expect interpreters to have a working knowledge of a range of subjects to the level expected when working in the higher education setting. Lecturers come to the classroom with a knowledge of the subject that they wish to transmit to the students, and their mind is working in a way that is linked to the subject matter. Interpreters, on the other hand, may have no knowledge of the subject, and come to it 'cold'. As the lecturer speaks, most of the students, who have followed the subject, hear the information directly from the source, and can follow the different tracks the lecturer may take. The interpreter also hears the information, but perhaps does not have background knowledge of the subject; nevertheless he or she has to translate this into BSL and convey it to the Deaf students as accurately as possible. The interpreter is not a lecturer, and does not have the same range or depth of knowledge, yet the students rely on him or her totally for subject information during the lecture. While their hearing colleagues receive the information directly, following the lecturer's train of thought in his or her own words, the Deaf students see the information only after it has passed through the mind of the interpreter. This may be at a level beyond the interpreter's personal experience, using jargon or specialist vocabulary, or it may involve deeper concepts (Harrington, 2001).

Consequently it is essential to make preparation materials available for interpreters well in advance of the lecture to enable them to absorb it and to familiarize themselves with any areas of uncertainty. Institutions could also help by giving library access and borrowing rights to interpreters, to enable them to do their own background preparation. The situation varies in different universities: some employ interpreters as part of their student support services; others, however, rely entirely on freelance interpreters brought in only for the lectures. In the latter case, the interpreters have no opportunity to access literature about the subjects they have to interpret, and little time or opportunity to consult with lecturers over specific vocabulary and concepts. Linked to this is the question of payment, since freelance interpreters are paid hourly for the time they spend in the classroom, and are not paid for their preparation time.

Interpreters employed as a team may support each other, discuss subjects and lectures, devise strategies for dealing with difficult jargon – and, most importantly, they have the time and resources to do this. Freelance interpreters are more likely to be isolated, working in education between other assignments, and may have neither the time nor the opportunity for familiarizing themselves with the subject.

Relationship with students and lecturers

The relationship between the main participants in the classroom is important, and the Project Officers identified a number of aspects of this from the videotaped data.

It is important that the interpreter knows when to say 'I don't know'. Students often stop interpreters to seek clarification or confirmation that they have understood correctly. In many cases, rather than stop the lecturer and voice the student's question, the project team observed interpreters, perhaps due to lack of confidence, carry on interpreting and, in addition, attempt to incorporate an explanation, rather than interrupt the flow of the lecturer.

The Project Officers also observed a number of occasions where interpreters overstepped the limits of their role by offering an explanation of what a teacher was saying, instead of facilitating the student by voicing a question to the teacher. As a result, the teacher continued, unaware that the student had a question or that the interpreter was no longer interpreting. Similar confusion arose when the interpreter did not actually understand what the lecturer was saying, but again lacked the confidence to stop the lecturer for clarification; instead, they continued signing what they thought it meant, resulting in Deaf students missing, or misunderstanding what the lecturer was actually saying. Some of these misunderstandings were rectified only when they were fed back in later coursework.

In an academic environment, a sign language interpreter has to operate at a level of language above that of the average interpreting assignment, and also has to cope with subject-specific vocabulary and jargon. For this, a background knowledge of the subject is needed, but in reality there are too few interpreters with academic backgrounds currently working in educational settings. In spite of having good BSL skills, then, it could happen that an interpreter simply cannot understand the theories a lecturer is propounding; in this scenario, the student will not be receiving full information and not, therefore, gaining access to the same learning that the hearing students experience.

It is also important that the relationship between the student and the interpreter is appropriate to the classroom and the needs of the other participants, including the teacher. The Project Officers observed several occasions where overfamiliarity between the interpreter and the student impeded both the message (in terms of what the student was given in the interpretation), and the relationship between the student and the other participants. Deaf students may be accustomed to working with the same interpreter; they may even know that interpreter personally from the local Deaf Club; nonetheless, working-relationship boundaries must be adhered to. It is tempting to refer to the interpreter for advice and support; however, this is the responsibility of the lecturer, and seeking advice from the interpreter about the course or the lecture may undermine the lecturer's position. At the same time, other students may see the student-interpreter relationship in a negative light, which further alienates the Deaf student.

Working conditions

In the university setting, interpreters are likely to find themselves working in isolation. Lectures can last up to 2 hours, and an interpreter doing three 2-hour sessions, one after the other, functions far less effectively towards the end of the day than at the beginning. Project analysis of the performances of interpreters working alone in morning sessions, compared with the same interpreters working alone in the afternoon, showed that misunderstanding of lesson content on the part of the interpreter and miscommunication of information is more likely to occur later in the day.

Fatigue will affect an interpreter's performance, and, working alone without a break, an interpreter is likely to function less effectively. The lecturer speaks, and the hearing audience receives his or her thoughts directly; the interpreter has to process those thoughts and translate them into BSL before conveying them to the Deaf students. Many lecturers are unaware of the language-processing functions carried out by the interpreter, and may not know to make allowances for time-lag or for the interpreter to catch up. This in itself is stressful; working alone adds to this and further reduces efficiency.

The environment can also have an impact on the interpreter's ability to function effectively. For example, on occasions, larger lecture theatres were poorly lit, particularly when OHPs or other visual media were being used; in some cases, Deaf students were unable to see the interpreter at all when rooms were 'blacked-out' for showing slides, yet lecturers continued speaking. Smaller teaching rooms were sometimes so cramped that the interpreter was sitting far too close to the student for comfort. Both interpreter and student felt uncomfortable if the signing-space was insufficient to allow for good communication. Focusing on an interpreter sitting too close affected understanding for the student, and the interpreter felt unable to sign effectively in cramped conditions. At other times the seating was set out in such a way that the interpreter was on the far side of the room, away from the lecturer and therefore unable to hear clearly what he or she was saying. All of this suggested that timetabling lectures in the most appropriate rooms would help increase the effectiveness of interpreted classes.

Co-working

When interpreters were co-working, analysis showed that this was not always effective. These situations could be improved in the following ways:

- Co-workers need to be free to decide whether to sit opposite each other or side by side, depending on the particular demands of any given setting, so they can support each other appropriately.
- The 'resting' interpreter should not leave the room, read or otherwise ignore the lesson while the other interpreter is on duty.
- The 'resting' interpreter should use appropriate and agreed strategies to feed the working interpreter with information he or she might have missed.
- Both interpreters should agree to use common vocabulary, and to watch each other to ensure that this happens.

Conclusion

This has been the first ever-British research project looking at the complex environment in which Deaf students have to study. It has recorded many hours of interpreted lectures, and has examined the complexities of the interaction between lecturers, interpreters and Deaf and hearing students. In the process, much has been revealed about the extent to which students may or may not effectively access education through interpreted teaching, and it has raised many interesting issues.

Among these is the question of responsibility: whose responsibility is it to ensure that Deaf students have equal access to learning? In the process of simultaneous translation, the interpreter must adapt and decode from one language – spoken English – to another – BSL; during this process, it is always possible that something vital may be lost in translation. Within the university environment, the level of language is academic and the theories often difficult to translate; it is essential that interpreters understand what is being said, and have adequate information and preparation from the lecturer to allow for effective interpretation. Of course, there is also a responsibility on the lecturer and students. Lecturers have to take ultimate responsibility for the content and clarity of their teaching; students, both Deaf and hearing, have to take responsibility for their own learning. It could be that the interpreting process makes this a more difficult task for Deaf students, which is why awareness, preparation and cooperation are all essential elements of the working relationships that have to exist between all of the participants in these settings.

During the project it was found that many universities used interpreters on a freelance basis, with their fees paid through individual students' DSA; the student, not the university, was in fact the interpreter's employer, though the arrangement was set up and facilitated by the university. This left interpreters unemployed or alternatively employed for half of the year but overworked during the two university semesters, with a comparatively low rate of pay and a great deal of anxiety. The solution may be for universities to offer interpreters secure contracts, within which they could be offered support, advice and training to enable them to work effectively at higher education level. It would perhaps be unrealistic to aim to employ all the interpreters needed to cope with the increasing demand brought about by an ever-increasing population of Deaf students, but a core of motivated and respected interpreters might support a 'bank' of freelancers.

In light of the outcomes of this project, such a system has been adopted by UCLAN, where the library-based SLRU operates an interpreting team lead by highly qualified and experienced academic interpreters. There is plenty for the employed interpreters to do during the 'idle' months from May to August, with the translation of texts on to BSL video and the preparation of resources in collaboration with academic departments and tutors. This apparently 'spare' time is also used for interpreter training and development. The findings of the Project have been very valuable and interesting and will continue to influence developments in the UCLAN and beyond.

References

Adolphs R (2002) How the brain processes emotional and social stimuli. London: British Neuropsychiatry Association Annual Meeting February 2002.

Ahmad W (ed) (1993) 'Race' and Health in Contemporary Britain. Buckingham: Open University Press.

Ahmad W, Atkin K (eds) (1996) 'Race' and Community Care. Buckingham: Open University Press.

Ahmad W, Darr A, Jones L, Nisar G (1998) Deafness and Ethnicity: services, policy and politics. West Sussex: Polity Press.

Albertini J (2000) Advances in literacy research and practice. Journal of Deaf Studies and Deaf Education 5(1): 123.

Allen C, Nikolopoulos TP, Dyar D, O'Donoghue GM (2001) The reliability of a rating scale for measuring speech intelligibility following pediatric cochlear implantation. Otology and Neurology 22: 631–633.

Allen C, Nikolopoulos TP, O'Donoghue G (1998) Speech intelligibility in children following cochlear implantation. American Journal of Otology 19(6): 742–746.

Anderson A, Bader M, Bard E, Boyle E, Doherty G, Garrod S, Isard S, Kowtko J, MacAllister J, Miller J, Sotillo C, Thompson H, Weinert R (1991) The HCRC map task corpus. Language and Speech 34: 351–366.

Archbold SM (1994) Developing a paediatric programme. In: McCormick B, Sheppard S, Archbold S (eds) Cochlear Implants in Young Deaf Children. London: Whurr.

Archbold SM Robinson K (1997) The European perspective on paediatric cochlear implantation, rehabilitation services and the educational implications. American Journal of Otology, 18: s75–s78.

Archbold SM, Lutman M, Marshall D (1995) Categories of auditory performance. Annals of Otology, Rhinology and Laryngology 104(suppl. 166): 312–314.

Archbold SM, Lutman ME, Nikolopoulos TP (1998) Categories of auditory performance: inter-user reliability. British Journal of Audiology 32: 7–12.

Archbold SM, O'Donoghue GM, Nikolopoulos TP (1998) Cochlear implants in children: an analysis of use over a 3-year period. American Journal of Otology, 19: 328–331.

Archbold SM, Nikolopoulos TP, O' Donoghue GM, Lutman ME (1998) Educational placement of deaf children following cochlear implantation. British Journal of Audiology 32: 295–300.

Archbold SM, Nikolopoulos TP, Lutman ME, ODonoghue GM (2002) The educational settings of profoundly deaf children with cochlear implants compared with age-matched hearing peers: implications for management. International Journal of Audiology 42(3): 157–161.

Archbold SM, Lutman ME, Gregory S, O'Neill C, Nikolopoulos TP (2002) Parents and their deaf child: their perceptions three years after cochlear implantation. Deafness and Education International 4(1): 12–40.

Atkinson JM, Heritage J (eds) (1984) Structures of Social Action. Studies in Conversation Analysis. Cambridge: Cambridge University Press.

Baker C (2000) The Care and Education of Young Bilinguals. An introduction for professionals. Clevedon: Multilingual Matters.

Baker P, Eversley J (eds) (2000) Multilingual Capital: The languages of London's schoolchildren and their relevance to economic, social and educational policies. London: Battlebridge Publications.

Baker R (1994) ESOL for adult deaf learners: Thoughts on the analysis and correction of errors. LASERBEAM 23: 21–25.

Bamford J, McCracken W, Peers I, Grayson P (1999) Trial of a two-channel hearing aid (low frequency compression-high-frequency linear amplification) with school age children. Ear and Hearing 20(4): 290–298.

Barnes D (1969) Language in the secondary classroom. In: Barnes D, Britton J, Rosen H (eds) Language, the Learner and the School. Harmondsworth: Penguin Education.

Barnes L (1996) Higher education and the deaf student: widening access or limiting participation. Paper given at 'The Dilemmas of Mass Higher Education, International Conference', Staffordshire University, 10 April 1996.

Barton ME, Strosberg R (1997) Conversational patterns of two-year-old twins in mother–twin–twin triads. Journal of Child Language 24, 257–269.

Barton ME, Tomasello M (1991) Joint attention and conversation in mother–infant–sibling triads. Child Development 62: 517–529.

Barton ME, Tomasello M (1994) The rest of the family: the role of fathers and siblings in early language development. In: Gallaway C, Richards BJ (eds) Input and Interaction in Language Acquisition. Cambridge: Cambridge University Press.

BDA (1996) The Right To Be Equal. London: British Deaf Association.

Belsky J, Cassidy J (1994) Attachment. In: Rutter M, Hay D (eds) Development Through Life. Oxford: Blackwell Scientific.

Berg F (1997) Listening learning environments. In: McCracken W, Laoide-Kemp S (eds.) Audiology in Education. London: Whurr.

Bernstein-Ratner N (1988) Patterns of parental vocabulary selection in speech to very young children. Journal of Child Language 15: 481–492.

Biering-Sorensen M, Riess H, Boisen G, Parving A (1995) A clinical comparative investigation of a non-linear versus linear hearing aid. Scandinavian Audiology 24: 125–132.

Blackledge A (2000) Literacy, Power and Social Justice. Stoke-on-Trent: Trentham Books.

Boothroyd A (1995) Speech perception tests and hearing impaired children. In: Plant G, Spens KE (eds) Profound Deafness and Speech Communication. London: Whurr.

Bornstein MH, Bruner JS (eds) (1989) Interaction in Human Development. Mahwah, NJ: Lawrence Erlbaum Associates.

Bornstein MH, Selmi AM, Haynes OM, Painter KM, Marx ES (1999) Representational abilities and the hearing status of child/mother dyads. Child Development 70(4): 833–852.

Bouvet D (1990) The Path to Language. Clevedon: Multilingual Matters.

Braungart-Rieker J, Courtney S, Garwood MM (1999) Mother– and father–infant attachment: families in context. Journal of Family Psychology 13(4): 535–553.

Brunved PB (1994) How studying loudness growth led to the development of Multifocus. Hearing Instruments 45: 8–10.

BSA (2001) The Adult Literacy Core Curriculum. London: Basic Skills Agency.

Burley S, Gutkin T, Naumann W (1994) Assessing the efficacy of an academic hearing peer tutor for a profoundly deaf student. American Annals of the Deaf 139: 415–419.

CACDP (2000) Certificate in Electronic Note-taking for Deaf People: Level 2 Curriculum. Durham: Council for the Advancement of Communication with Deaf People.

CACDP (2001) Code of Practice for Communication Support Workers. Durham: Council for the Advancement of Communication with Deaf People.

Caissie R, Wilson E (1995) Communication breakdown management during co-operative learning activities by mainstreamed students with hearing losses. Volta Review 97: 105–121.

Campbell R (1996) Guest Editorial. Journal of Deaf Studies and Deaf Education 1(4): 215–216.

Chalmers R (1996) Sylheti: a regional language of Bangladesh. European Network of Bangladeshi Studies – E.C. Research Paper #5/5–96. Bath: Institute of Development Studies, University of Bath.

Chamba R, Ahmad W, Jones L (1998) Improving Services for Asian Deaf Children. Bristol: Policy Press.

Charrow VR, Fletcher JD (1974) English as the second language of deaf children. Developmental Psychology 10(4): 463–470.

Cheng AK, Grant GD, Niparko JK (1999) Meta-analysis of pediatric cochlear implant literature. Annals of Otology, Rhinology and Laryngology Suppl 117: 124–128.

Chiat S (2000) Understanding Children with Language Problems. Cambridge: Cambridge University Press.

CICHS (1995) Speech and language therapy services for bilingual clients in Camden and Islington: proposed service developments and issues of equal access. London: Clinical Audit Department, Camden and Islington Community Health Services NHS Trust.

Clibbens J (1998) ESRC Cognition and Deafness Seminar No 3: Report. Deafness and Education 22(2): 61–62.

Cline T (1998) The assessment of special educational needs for bilingual children. British Journal of Special Education 25(4): 159–163.

Conrad R (1979) The Deaf Schoolchild: Language and Cognitive Function. New York: Harper & Row.

Cooper CR, Marquis A, Edward D (1986) Four perspectives on peer learning among elementary school children. In: Mueller EC, Cooper CR (eds) Process and Outcome in Peer Relationships. Orlando, FL: Academic Press.

Corrin J, Tarplee C, Wells B (2001) Interactional linguistics and languiage development: a conversation analytic perspective on emergent syntax.

In: Couper-Kuhlen E, Selting M (eds) Studies in Interactional Linguistics. Amsterdam: Benjamins.

Courtin C (2000) The impact of sign language on the cognitive development of deaf children: the case of theories of mind. Journal of Deaf Studies and Deaf Education 5(3): 266–276.

Courtin C, Melot A-M (1998) Development of theories of mind in deaf children. In Marschark M, Clark MC (eds) Psychological Perspectives on Deafness: vol. 2. Mahwah, NJ: Lawrence Erlbaum Associates.

Cox R, Alexander G (1991) Hearing aid benefit in everyday environments. Ear and Hearing 12(2): 127–139.

Cox R, Alexander G (1995) The abbreviated profile of hearing aid benefit. Ear and Hearing 16(2):176–186.

Cullen R (1998) Teacher talk and the classroom context. English Language and Teaching Journal 52(3): 179–187.

Cumming A (1987) Writing expertise and second language proficiency in ESL writing performance. Unpublished doctoral dissertation, University of Toronto.

Cunningham-Andersson U, Andersson S (1999) Growing Up with Two Languages: a practical guide. London: Routledge.

Daniels S, Corlett S (1990) Deaf Students in Higher Education: A survey of policy and practice. RNID Research Report No.9, London: RNID.

Davidson RG, Snow CE (1996) Five-year-olds' interactions with fathers versus mothers. First Language 16: 223–242.

De Houwer A (1995) Bilingual language acquisition. In: Fletcher P, MacWhinney B (eds) The Handbook of Child Language. Oxford: Blackwell.

DfEE (1998) The National Literacy Strategy: framework for teaching. London: HMSO.

DfEE (2000) Draft Revised Code of Practice for Special Educational Needs. London: The Stationery Office.

DfEE (2001a) URL *http://vtc.ngfl.gov.uk/literacy/nls/eal.html*.

DfEE (2001b) URL: *http://www.dfee.gov.uk/ethnic/guide.htm*.

Dillon H (1996) Compression? Yes but for low or high frequencies, for low or high intensities and with what response times? Ear and Hearing 17: 287–307.

Dillon H (2001) Hearing Aids. New York: Thieme.

Dillon H, Ching T (1995) Tests of speech perception. In Plant G, Spens KE (eds). Profound Deafness and Speech Communication. London: Whurr.

Diniz FA (1999) Race and special education needs in the 1990s. British Journal of Special Education 26(4): 213–217.

Dinsmore DJ (1985) Waiting for Godot in the EFL classroom. English Language Teaching Journal 39(4): 225–234.

Doise W, Mugny G (1984) The Social Development of the Intellect. Oxford: Pergamon.

Drasgow E (1993) Bilingual/bicultural education: an overview. Sign Language Studies 80: 243–265.

Drew P (1990) Conversation analysis. In: Asher RE, Simpson JMY (eds) The Encyclopaedia of Language and Linguistics. Oxford: Pergamon.

Dromi E, Ingber S (1999) Israeli mothers' expectations from early intervention with their preschool deaf children. Journal of Deaf Studies and Deaf Education 4(1): 50–68.

Dunn J (1996) The Emmanuel Miller Memorial Lecture 1995. Children's relationships: Bridging the divide between cognitive and social development. Journal of Child Psychology and Psychiatry 37: 507–518.

Dunn J, Kendrick C (1982) The speech of 2- and 3-year olds to infant siblings: 'baby talk' and the context of communication. Journal of Child Language 9: 579–595.

Durkin K (1995) Developmental Social Psychology: From Infancy to Old Age. Oxford: Blackwell.

Dyar D (1994) Monitoring Progress: The Role of a Speech and Language Therapist. In: McCormick B, Archbold S, Sheppard S (eds) (1994) Cochlear Implants for Young Children. London: Whurr.

Easterbrooks SR (1998). Encouraging conversation: teachers and students talking together. Volta Voices 5(3): 20–21.

Edelsky C (1982) Writing in a bilingual program: The relation of L1 and L2 texts. TESOL Quarterly 16(2): 211–229.

Edelsky C, Jilbert K (1985). Bilingual children and writing: lessons for all of us. Volta Review 87(5): 57–72.

Edinburgh Reading Test (1977) London: Hodder and Stoughton.

Edwards V (1998) The Tower of Babel: Teaching and learning in multilingual classrooms. Stoke-on-Trent: Trentham Books.

Egan D (1988) Architectural Acoustics. New York: McGraw Hill.

Elliot L, Stinson M, McKee B, Everhart V, Francis P (2001) College students' perceptions of the C-Print speech to text transcription system, Journal of Deaf Studies and Deaf Education 6(4): 285–298.

Ellis S, Rogoff B (1986) Problem solving in children's management of instruction. In Mueller EC, Cooper CR (eds) (1986) Process and Outcome in Peer Relationships. Orlando, FL: Academic Press.

Everhart VS, Marschark M (1988) Linguistic flexibility in the written and signed/oral language productions of deaf and hearing children. Journal of Experimental Child Psychology 46: 174–193.

Fairclough N (1992) Discourse and Social Change. Cambridge: Polity Press.

Fernald A, Morikawa H (1993) Common themes and cultural variations in Japanese and American's speech to infants. Child Development 64: 637–656.

Flavell JH, Miller PH (1998) Social cognition. In: Kuhn D, Siegler RS (eds.) Handbook of Child Psychology: cognition, perception and language, Vol.2, 5th edn. New York: Wiley.

Fletcher P, MacWhinney B (eds) (1995) The Handbook of Child Language. Oxford: Blackwell.

Fletcher-Campbell, F (1992) How can we use an extra pair of hands? British Journal of Special Education 19 (4): 141–143.

Fortnum HM, Marshall DH, Bamford JM, Summerfield AQ (2002) Hearing-impaired children in the UK: education setting and communication approach. Deafness and Education International 4 (3): 123–141.

Foster S, Long G, Snell K (1999) Inclusive instruction and learning for deaf students in postsecondary education. Journal of Deaf Studies and Deaf Education 4(3): 225–235.

Francis HW, Koch ME, Wyatt JR, Niparko JK (1999) Trends in educational placement and cost-benefit considerations in children with cochlear implants. Archives of Otolaryngology, Head and Neck Surgery 125: 499–505.

Francis N (1999) Bilingualism, writing, and metalinguistic awareness: oral-literate interactions between first and second languages. Applied Psycholinguistics 20: 533–561.

Freeman RD, Malkin SF, Hastings JO (1975) Psycho-social problems of deaf children and their families: A comparative study. American Annals of the Deaf 120: 391–405.

Friedlander A (1990) Composing in English: effects of first language on writing in English as a second language. In: Kroll B (ed) Second Language Writing. Cambridge: Cambridge University Press.

Fryauf-Bertschy H, Tyler R, Kelsay DMR, Gantz BJ, Woodworth GG (1997) Cochlear implant use by prelingually deafened children: the influence of age at implant and length of device use. Journal of Speech Language and Hearing Research 40: 183–199.

Gallaway C, Hostler ME, Reeves D (1990) Speech addressed to hearing-impaired children by their mothers. Clinical Linguistics and Phonetics 4(3): 221–237.

Gallaway C, Richards BJ (eds) (1994). Input and Interaction in Language Acquisition. Cambridge: Cambridge University Press.

Gallaway C, Woll B (1994) Interaction and childhood deafness. In: Gallaway C, Richards BJ (eds) Input and Interaction in Language Acquisition. Cambridge: Cambridge University Press.

Garner PW (1996) The relations of emotional role taking, affective/moral attributions, and emotional display rule knowledge to low-income school-age children's social competence. Journal of Applied Developmental Psychology 17: 19–36.

Gatehouse S (1993) Role of perceptual acclimatization in the selection of frequency responses for hearing aids. Journal of the American Academy of Audiology 4: 296–306.

Geekie P, Raban B (1994) Language learning at home and at school. In: Gallaway C, Richards BJ (eds) Input and Interaction in Language Acquisition. Cambridge: Cambridge University Press.

Glaser B, Strauss A (1967) The Discovery of Grounded Theory. Chicago, IL: Aldine.

Gleason JB (1975) Fathers and other strangers: men's speech to young children. In: Dato D (ed) Developmental Psycholinguistics: theory and applications. Washington, DC: Georgetown University Press.

Goldberg J, Bordman P (1975) The ESL approach to teaching English to hearing impaired students. American Annals of the Deaf 120: 22–27.

Goodman R, Meltzer H, Bailey V (1998) The strengths and difficulties questionnaire: A pilot study on the validity of the self-report version. European Child and Adolescent Psychiatry 7: 125–130.

Gray CD, Hosie JA, Russell PA, Ormel EA (2001) Emotion development in deaf children: facial expressions, display rules and theory of mind. In: Clark MD, Marschark M, Karchmer M (eds) Context, Cognition and Deafness. Washington, DC: Gallaudet University Press.

Green C, Nickerson W (1992) The Rise of the Communicator: a Perspective on Post-16 Education and Training for Deaf People. Chesterfield: Moonshine Books.

Greenberg MT (2000) Educational interventions: Prevention and promotion of competence. In: Hindley P, Kitson N (eds) Mental Health and Deafness. London: Whurr.

Greenberg MT, Kusché C (1993) Promoting Social and Emotional Development in Deaf Children: The PATHS Project. Seattle, WA: University of Washington Press.

Gregory E (1996) Making Sense of a New World – Learning to Read in a Second Language. London: Paul Chapman.

Gregory E (1998) Siblings as mediators of literacy in linguistic minority communities. Language and Education 12(1): 33–54.

Gregory S (1976) The Deaf Child and His Family. London: George Allen and Unwin.

Gregory S (1997) Deaf children's writing: The influence of British Sign Language on written English. Paper presented to the International Symposium on Bilingualism, University of Newcastle upon Tyne, April 1997.

Gregory S (2001) Psychosocial Issues. Paper presented at Cochlear Implantation: Cost Creating or Cost Saving? Nottingham, 18 May 2001.

Gregory S, Bishop J (1989). The education of deaf children into ordinary schools: a research report. Journal of the British Association of Teachers of the Deaf 13(1): 1–6.

Gregory S, Bishop J, Sheldon L (1995) Deaf Young People and Their Families. Cambridge: Cambridge University Press.

Gregory S, Knight P (1998) Social development and family life. In: Gregory S, Knight P, McCracken W, Powers S, Watson L (eds) Issues in Deaf Education. London: David Fulton.

Gregory S, Knight P, McCracken W, Powers S, Watson L (eds) (1998) Issues in Deaf Education. London: David Fulton.

Grimshaw, S (1996) The extraction of listening situations which are relevant to young children, and the perceptions of normal hearing subjects of the degree of difficulty experienced by the hearing impaired in different types of listening situations. Unpublished report, MRC Institute of Hearing Research.

Happé F, Frith U (1996) Theory of mind and social impairment in children with conduct disorder. British Journal of Developmental Psychology 14: 385–398.

Harrington FJ (2001) The rise, fall and reinvention of the communicator: redefining roles and responsibilities in educational interpreting. In: Harrington FJ, Turner GH (eds) Interpreting Interpreting: studies and reflections on sign language interpreting. Coleford, UK: Douglas McLean and *http://www.directlearn.co.uk/deafres.htm*.

Harris M (2000) Social interaction and early language development in deaf children. Deafness and Education International 2(1): 1–11.

Harrison MJ, Magill-Evans J, Sadoway D (2001) Scores on the Nursing Child Assessment Teaching Scale for father–toddler dyads. Public Health Nursing 18(2): 94–100.

Hawkins D, Naidoo S (1993) Comparison of sound quality and clarity with asymmetrical peak clipping and output limiting compression. Journal of American Academy of Audiology 4: 222–228.

HEFCE (1996) Access to Higher Education: students with learning difficulties and disabilities (A report on the 1993/4 and 1994/5 HEFCE special initiatives to encourage widening participation in higher education). London: Higher Education Funding Council for England.

Hehar SS, Nikolopoulos TP, Gibbin KP, O'Donoghue GM (2002) Surgery and functional outcomes in deaf children implanted under the age of two years. Archives of Otorhinolaryngology – Head and Neck Surgery 128: 11–14.

Herman R, Holmes S, Woll B (1999) BSL Language Development: Receptive Skills Test. Coelford: Forest Bookshop.

Hindley PA, Gent T van (2000). Mental health in deaf children and adolescents: an Anglo-Dutch collaborative study. Poster-presentation at the Fourth European Conference of the Association for Child Psychology and Psychiatry, London.

Hindley PA (2000) Child and Adolescent Psychiatry. In: Hindley P, Kitson N (eds.) Mental Health and Deafness. London: Whurr.

Hindley PA, Reed H (1999) Promoting Alternative Thinking Strategies (PATHS): mental health promotion with deaf children in school. In Decker S, Kirby S, Greenwood A, Moore D (eds.) Taking Children Seriously: applications of counselling and therapy in education. London: Cassell.

Hintermair M (2000) Hearing impairment, social networks and coping: The need for families with hearing impaired children to relate to other parents and to hearing-impaired adults. American Annals of the Deaf 145: 41–51.

Hladik EG, Edwards HT (1984) A comparative analysis of mother–father speech in the naturalistic home environment. Journal of Psycholinguistic Research 13: 321–332.

HMSO (1989) The Children Act, 1989. London: HMSO.

HMSO (1992) Further and Higher Education Act. London: HMSO.

HMSO (1995) Disability Discrimination Act (Chapter 50) London: HMSO.

Hoffmann C (1991) An Introduction to Bilingualism. London: Longman.

Hoffmeister RJ, Shettle C (1981) Results of a family sign language intervention program. Paper presented at 50th Meeting of the Convention of American Instructors of the Deaf, Rochester, NY.

Hopwood V (2000). The effect of teaching context on language interaction with deaf pupils in mainstream schools. PhD Thesis, University of Manchester.

Hopwood V, Gallaway C (1999). Evaluating the linguistic experience of a deaf child in a mainstream class: a case study. Deafness and Education International 1(3):172–187.

Howell DC (1992) Statistical Methods for Psychology, 3rd edn. Belmont, CA: Duxbury Press.

Hudelson S (1989) Write on: children writing in ESL. Englewoods Cliffs, NJ: Prentice Hall.

Hurst A (1993) Steps Towards Graduation. Avebury: Aldershot and Brookefield.

Hutchby I, Wooffit R (1998) Conversation Analysis. Principles, practices and applications. Cambridge: Polity Press.

Jamieson JR (1994) Instructional discourse strategies: Differences between hearing and deaf mothers of deaf children. First Language 14: 153–171.

Jeanes RC, Nienhuys TGWM, Rickards FW (2000) The pragmatic skills of profoundly deaf children. Journal of Deaf Studies and Deaf Education 5: 237–247.

Johnson HA, Griffith PL (1986) The instructional patterns of two fourth-grade spelling classes: a mainstreaming issue. American Annals of the Deaf 131 (5): 331–338.

Johnson K (1992) Miscommunication in interpreted classroom interaction. In Cokely D (ed) Sign Language Interpreters and Interpreting. Burtonsville, MD: Linstock Press.

Jones P (1979) Negative interference of signed language in written English. Sign Language Studies 24: 273–279.

Kampfe CM, Harrison M, Oettinger T, Ludington J, McDonald-Bell C, Pillsbury HC 3d (1993) Parental expectations as a factor in evaluating children for the multichannel cochlear implant. American Annals of the Deaf 138(3): 297–303.

Kelsay DM, Tyler RS (1996) Advantages and disadvantages expected and realized by pediatric cochlear implant recipients as reported by their parents. American Journal of Otology 17(6): 866–73.

Kluwin TN (1985) The acquisition of content from a signed lecture. Sign Language Studies 48: 269–286.

Knight P (1997) Bilingual nursery provision: a challenging start. Deafness and Education (Journal of the British Association of Teachers of the Deaf) 21(3): 20–30.

Kopun JG, Stelmachowicz PG (1998) Perceived communication difficulties in children with hearing loss. American Journal of Audiology 7: 30–37.

Krapels A (1990). An overview of second language writing process research. In: Kroll B (ed) Second Language Writing. Cambridge: Cambridge University Press.

Kretschmer R, Kretschmer L (1995). Communication-based classrooms. Volta Review 97(5) (monograph): 1–18.

Lane H (1995) Letter to the editor. American Journal of Otology 16(3): 393–399.

Lane H, Bahan B (1998) Ethics of cochlear implantation in young deaf children: a review and reply from a Deaf-World perspective. Otolaryngology, Head and Neck Surgery 119(4): 297–313.

Lane H, Hoffmeister R, Bahan B (1996) A journey into the Deaf-World. San Diego, CA: DawnSign Press.

Lau A (ed) (2000) South Asian Children and Adolescents in Britain: Ethno-cultural issues. London: Whurr.

Lawrence RF, Moore BCJ, Glasberg BR (1983) A comparison of behind-the-ear high-fidelity linear hearing aids and two channel compression hearing aids. Audiology 17: 31–48.

Leather C, Wirz S (1996) Centre for International Child Health: The training and development needs of bilingual support workers in the NHS in community settings. London: NHS Executive, Department of Health.

Lederberg AR, Everhart VS (2000) Conversations between deaf children and their hearing mothers: pragmatic and dialogic characteristics. Journal of Deaf Studies and Deaf Education 5(4): 303–310.

Levinson SC (1983) Pragmatics. Cambridge: Cambridge University Press.

Lichtenstein E (1998) The relationships between reading processes and English skills of deaf college students. Journal of Deaf Studies and Deaf Education 3(2): 80–134.

Lieven EVM (1994) Crosslinguistic and crosscultural aspects of language addressed to children. In: Gallaway C, Richards BJ (eds) Input and Interaction in Language Acquisition. Cambridge: Cambridge University Press.

Light P, Littleton K (1999) Social Processes in Children's Learning. Cambridge: Cambridge University Press.

Lloyd J (1999a) Interaction between hearing-impaired children and their normally hearing peers. Deafness and Education International 1: 25–33.

Lloyd J (1999b) Hearing-impaired children's strategies for managing communication breakdowns. Deafness and Education International 1: 188–199.

Lloyd J, Lieven E, Arnold P (2001) Oral conversations between hearing-impaired children and their normally hearing peers and teachers. First Language 21: 83–107.

Lloyd P (1991) Strategies used to communicate route directions by telephone: a comparison of the performance of 7-year-olds, 10-year-olds and adults. Journal of Child Language 18: 171–189.

Lloyd P (1992) The role of clarification requests in children's communication of route directions by telephone. Discourse Processes 15: 357–374.

Lloyd P (1993) Referential communication as teaching: Adults tutoring their own and other children. First Language 13: 339–357.

Lundy JEB (2002) Age and language skills of deaf children in relation to theory of mind development. Journal of Deaf Studies and Deaf Education 7 (1): 41–56.

Lynas W (1986) Integrating the Handicapped into Ordinary Schools. Beckenham: Croom Helm.

Lynas W (1999a) Supporting the deaf child in the mainstream school: is there a best way? Support for Learning 14 (3): 113–121.

Lynas W (1999b) Identifying effective practice: a study of the educational achievements of a small sample of profoundly deaf children. Deafness and Education International 1 (3): 155–171.

Lynas W, Lewis S, Hopwood V (1997) Supporting the education of deaf children in mainstream schools. Deafness and Education 21: 41–45.

Lyon M (1985) The verbal interaction of mothers and their preschool hearing-impaired children: a preliminary investigation. Journal of the British Association for Teachers of the Deaf 9(5): 119–129.

McCarthy M (1991) Discourse Analysis for Language Teachers. Cambridge: Cambridge University Press.

McLaughlin B, White D, McDevitt T, Raskin R (1983) Mothers' and fathers' speech to their young children: similar or different? Journal of Child Language 10: 245–252.

McLoughlin M (1987) A history of the education of the deaf. Liverpool: McLoughlin.

McNamara S (1997) Children with special educational needs: Supporting the learning relationship. In: Kitson N, Merry R (eds) Teaching in the Primary School: a learning relationship. London: Routledge, pp. 65–84.

MacSweeney M (1998) Cognition and deafness. In: Gregory S, Knight P, McCracken W, Powers S, Watson L (eds) Issues in Deaf Education. London: David Fulton.

Mahon M (1997) Conversational interactions between young deaf children and their families in homes where English is not the first language. Unpublished PhD Thesis, University College London.

Mannle S, Barton M, Tomasello M (1991) Two-year-olds' conversations with their mothers and preschool-aged siblings. First Language 12: 57–71.

Markides A (1986) Speech levels and speech-to-noise ratios. British Journal of Audiology 20: 115–120.

Martinez MA (1987) Dialogues among children and between children and their mothers. Child Development 58: 1035–1043.

Masur EF, Gleason JB (1980) Parent–child interaction and the acquisition of lexical information during play. Developmental Psychology 16: 404–409.

Mayer C (1999) Shaping at the point of utterance: An investigation of the composing processes of the deaf student writer. Journal of Deaf Studies and Deaf Education 4(1): 37–49.

Mayer C, Akamatsu CT (2000). Deaf children creating written texts: contributions of American sign language and signed forms of English. American Annals of the Deaf, 145 (5): 394–403.

Mayer C, Wells G (1996) Can the linguistic interdependence theory support a bilingual-bicultural model of literacy education for deaf students? Journal of Deaf Studies and Deaf Education 1(2): 93–107.

Mellon N (2000) Language acquisition. In: Niparko J, Iler Kirk K, Mellon NK, McConkey Robbins A, Tucci D L, Wilson BS (eds) (2000) Cochlear Implants: Principles and Practice. Philadelphia, PA: Lippincott Williams & Wilkins.

Meltzer H, Gatward R with Goodman R, Ford T (2000) The Mental Health of Children and Adolescents in Great Britain. London: Office for National Statistics.

Mercer N (1992) Talk for teaching and learning. In: Norman K (ed.) Thinking Voices: the work of the National Oracy Project. London: Hodder and Stoughton.

Mertens D (1991) Teachers working with interpreters: the deaf student's educational experience. American Annals of the Deaf 136: 48–52.

Miller AL, Vollig BL, McElwain NL (2000) Sibling jealousy in a triadic context with mothers and fathers. Social Development 9(4): 433–457.

Miller KJ (1995) Co-operative conversations: The effect of co-operative learning in conversational interaction. American Annals of the Deaf 140(1): 28–37.

Mittler P (1989) Foreword: Towards education for all. In Webster A, Wood D. Children with Hearing Difficulties. London: Cassell.

Miyamoto RT, Kirk KI, Todd SL, Robbins AM, Osberger MJ (1995) Speech perception skills of children with multichannel cochlear implants of hearing aids. Annals of Otology, Rhinology and Laryngology 104(suppl 166): 334–337.

Miyamoto RT, Svirsky MA, Robbins AM (1997) Enhancement of expressive language in prelingually deaf children with cochlear implants. Acta Otolaryngologica 117(2): 154–157.

Mohay H (2000) Language in sight: mothers' strategies for making language visually accessible to deaf children. In: Spencer PE, Erting CJ, Marschark M (eds) The Deaf Child in the Family and at School. London: Lawrence Erlbaum Associates.

Mohay H, Milton L, Hindmarsh G, Ganley K (1998) Deaf mothers as language models for hearing families with deaf children. In: Weisel A (ed.) Issues Unresolved: new perspectives on language and deafness. Washington, DC: Gallaudet University Press.

Monkman H, Baskind S (1998) Are assistants effectively supporting hearing impaired children in mainstream schools? Deafness and Education (Journal of the British Association of Teachers of the Deaf) 22(1): 15–22.

Moog JS, Geers AE (1999) Speech and language acquisition in young children after cochlear implantation. Otolaryngologic Clinics of North America 32(6): 1127–1141.

Moore BCJ (1995) Perceptual Consequences of Cochlear Damage. Oxford: Oxford University Press.

Moore BCJ, Glasberg BR (1986) A comparison of two-channel and single-channel compression aids. Audiology 25: 210–226.

Moore BCJ, Johnson JS, Clark TN, Pluvinage, V (1992) A comparison of four implementing automatic gain control (AGC) in hearing aids. British Journal of Audiology 22: 93–104.

Moseley D (1976) Helping with Learning Difficulties. Course E201 OU: Block 10. Milton Keynes: Open University.

Mozzer-Mather S (1990). A strategy to improve deaf students' writing through the use of glosses of signed narratives. Gallaudet Research Institute Working paper 90–4. Washington, DC: Gallaudet University.

Musselman C (2000) How do children who can't hear learn to read an alphabetic script? A review of the literature on reading and deafness. Journal of Deaf Studies and Deaf Education 5(1): 9–31.

Musselman C, Churchill A (1992) The effects of maternal conversational control on deaf children: a longitudinal study. Journal of Childhood Communication Disorders 14: 99–118.

Musselman C, Churchill A (1993) Maternal control and the development of deaf children: a test of the stage hypothesis. First Language 13:271–290.

Musselman C, Hambleton D (1990). Creating classroom conversations with deaf children. ACEHI Journal/la Revue ACEDA16 (2–3): 68–90.

Naeem Z, Newton V (1996) Prevalence of sensori-neural hearing loss in Asian children. British Journal of Audiology 30(5): 332–339.

Nakisa MJ, Summerfield AQ, Nakisa RC, McCormick B, Archbold S, Gibbin KP, O'Donoghue GM (2001) Functionally equivalent ages and hearing levels of children with cochlear implants measured with pre-recorded stimuli. British Journal of Audiology 35: 183–199.

NALDIC (2001) URL: *http://www.naldic.org.uk/*

NATED (2002) Assessment Pack, 2nd edn. New College, Redditch: National Association for Tertiary Education for Deaf People.

NDCS(1996) Quality Standards in Paediatric Audiology – Volume II. London: National Deaf Children's Society.

NDCS (1999) PATHS: A report on the NDCS deaf children in mind project – a personal social initiative. London: National Deaf Children's Society.

Neuroth-Gimbrone C, Logiodice CM (1992). A co-operative bilingual language programme for deaf adolescents. Sign Language Studies 74: 79–91.

Nikolopoulos TP, Archbold SM, O'Donoghue GM (1999) The development of auditory perception in children following cochlear implantation. International Journal of Pediatric Otorhinolaryngology 49(suppl.1): 189–191.

Nikolopoulos TP, O'Donoghue GM, Archbold SM (1999) Age at implantation: Its importance in paediatric cochlear implantation. Laryngoscope 109: 595–599.

Nikolopoulos TP, Wells P, Archbold SM (2000) Using Listening Progress Profile (LIP) to assess early functional auditory performance in young implanted children. Deafness and Education International 2(3): 142–151.

Nikolopoulos TP, Archbold SM, Lutman ME, O'Donoghue G (2000) Prediction of auditory performance following cochlear implantation of prelingually deaf young children. In: Waltzman SB, Cohen NL (eds) Cochlear Implants. New York: Thieme Medical Publishers.

Nikolopoulos TP, Dyar D, Archbold SM, O'Donoghue GM (in press) Development of spoken language grammar in prelingually deaf children following cochlear implantation. Laryngoscope.

Nikolopoulos TP, Lloyd H, Archbold SM, O'Donoghue GM (2001) Pediatric cochlear implantation: the parents' perspective. Archives of Otorhinolaryngology – Head and Neck Surgery 127: 363–367.

Niver JM, Schery TK (1994) Deaf children's spoken language output with a hearing peer and with a hearing mother. American Annals of the Deaf 139: 96–103.

Nottingham Paediatric Cochlear Implant Programme (undated) Brochure. Available from NPCIP, Ropewalk House, 113 The Ropewalk, Nottingham NG1 6HA, UK.

Nunan D (1987) Communicative language teaching: making it work. English Language Teaching Journal 41(2): 136–145.

O'Donoghue GM, Nikolopoulos TP, Archbold SM (2000) Determinants of speech perception in children after cochlear implantation. Lancet 356(9228): 466–468.

O'Donoghue GM, Nikolopoulos TP, Archbold SM, Tait M (1998) Speech perception in children following cochlear implantation. American Journal of Otology 19(6): 762–767.

Office of National Statistics (2001) URL: *http://www.statistics.gov.uk/statbase/xsdataset.asp*

Olsen J (1992) From acoustic amplification to hearing loss compensation. Hearing Instruments 43: 12–18.

Olson D (1996) The World on Paper: the conceptual and cognitive implications of writing and reading. Cambridge: Cambridge University Press.

O'Neill C, O'Donoghue GM, Archbold SM, Normand C (2000) A cost-utility analysis of paediatric cochlear implantation. Laryngoscope 110: 156–160.

O'Neill R, Mowat P, Gallagher J, Atkins P (2002) Deaf students and their support in further education in the United Kingdom – Results from the National Association for Tertiary Education for Deaf People Survey 2000, Deafness and Educational International 4(2): 99–114.

Palmer CV, Mormer EA (1999) Goals and expectations of hearing aid fittings. Trends in Amplification 4 (2): 61–71.

Pappas Jones C, Adamson LB (1987) Language use in mother–child and mother–child–sibling interactions. Child Development 58: 356–366.

Paul PV (1998) Literacy and Deafness: the development of reading, writing and literate thought. London: Allyn and Bacon.

Paul PV, Quigley P (2000) Language and Deafness, 3rd edn. San Diego, CA: College-Hill Press.

Peterson CC, Siegal M (1999) Representing inner worlds: theory of mind in autistic, deaf, and normal hearing children. Psychological Science 10: 126–129.

Peterson ME (1993) Fitting children with Multifocus hearing aids. Hearing Instruments 44: 33–35.

Peterson ME, Feeney P, Yantis PA (1990) The effect of AGC in hearing-impaired listeners with different dynamic ranges. Ear and Hearing 11: 185–194.

Petitto LA, Katerelos M, Levy BG, Gauna K, Tetreault K, Ferraro V (2001) Bilingual signed and spoken language acquisition from birth: implications for the mechanisms underlying early bilingual language acquisition. Journal of Child Language 28: 453–496.

Piaget J (1932) The Moral Judgement of the Child. London: Routledge.

Pickersgill M (1998) Bilingualism – current policy and practice. In: Gregory S, Knight P, McCracken W, Powers S, Watson L (eds) Issues in Deaf Education. London: David Fulton Publishers.

Pickersgill M, Gregory S (1998) Sign bilingualism. A model. Wembley: LASER.

Plapinger D, Kretschmer R (1991). The effect of context on the interactions between a normally-hearing mother and her hearing impaired child. Volta Review 93, 75–87.

Powers S (1990) A survey of secondary units for hearing impaired children. Journal of the British Association of Teachers of the Deaf 14(3): 69–79.

Powers S (1998) The educational attainments of deaf children. In: Gregory S, Knight P, McCracken W, Powers S, Watson L (eds) (1998) Issues in Deaf Education. London: David Fulton Publishers.

Powers S, Gregory S, Thoutenhoofd ED (1998) The educational achievements of deaf children; a literature review. Research Report 65. London: Dept for Education and Employment.

Pressman L, Pipp-Siegel S, Yoshinaga-Itano C, Deas A (1999) Maternal sensitivity predicts language gain in preschool children who are deaf and hard of hearing. Journal of Deaf Studies and Deaf Education 4(4): 294–301.

Prezbindowski AK, Adamson, LB, Lederberg AR (1998) Joint attention in deaf and hearing 22 month-old children and their hearing mothers. Journal of Applied Developmental Psychology 19(3): 377–387.

Radford J, Tarplee C (2000) The management of conversational topic by a ten-year-old child with pragmatic difficulties. Clinical Linguistics and Phonetics 14: 387–408.

Rawlinson S J (1998) The Americans with Disabilities Act: applications in post secondary education of students who are deaf/hard of hearing. Journal of Deaf Studies and Deaf Education 3(4): 339–340.

RCSLT (1998) Royal College of Speech and Language Therapists Specific Interest Group in Bilingualism. Good practice for speech and language therapists working with clients from linguistic minorities. London: Royal College of Speech and Language Therapists.

Reich C, Hambleton D, Houldin BK (1977). The integration of hearing impaired children in regular classrooms. American Annals of the Deaf 122: 534–543.

Remmel E, Bettger JG, Weinberg AM (2001) Theory of mind in deaf children. In: Clark MD, Marschark M, Karchmer M. (eds) Context, Cognition and Deafness. Washington, DC: Gallaudet University Press.

Richards BJ, Gallaway C (1994). Speech addressed to children. In Asher RE, Simpson JMY (eds) Encyclopaedia of Language Learning and Linguistics. Oxford: Pergamon Press.

Ridley J, Radford J, Mahon M (2002) How do teachers manage topic and repair? Child Language Teaching and Therapy 18: 43–59.

Ringdahl A, Eriksson-Mangold M, Anderson G (1998) Psychometric evaluation of the Gothenburg Profile for measurement of experienced hearing disability and handicap: applications with new hearing aid candidates and experienced hearing aid users. British Journal of Audiology 32: 75–385.

RNID (2001) Deaf Students in Further Education. Educational Guidelines Project, London: Royal National Institute for Deaf People.

RNID/NDCS (2000) Statement of Competencies for Working with Children 0–2 and their Families. London: Royal National Institute for Deaf People.

Roberts SB, Rickards FW (1994). A survey of graduates of an Australian integrated auditory/oral preschool. Part II: Academic achievement, utilisation of support services and friendship patterns. Volta Review 96(3): 207–236.

Robson C (1993) Real World Research. Oxford: Blackwell.

Rodda M, Eleweke J (2000) Theories of literacy development in deaf people with limited English proficiency. Deafness and Education International 2(2): 101–113.

Rogoff B (1990) Apprenticeship in Thinking: cognitive development in social context. New York: Oxford University Press.

Rogoff B (1991) The joint socialization of development by young children and adults. In: Light P, Sheldon S, Woodhead M (eds) Learning to Think. London: Routledge.

Romaine S (1994) Bilingualism, 2nd edn. Oxford: Blackwell.

Rondal JA (1980) Fathers' and mothers' speech in early language development. Journal of Child Language 7(2): 353–369.

Rose DE, Vernon N, Pool AF (1996) Cochlear implants in prelingually deaf children. American Annals of the Deaf 141: 258–261.

Roy CB (1993) A sociolinguistic analysis of the interpreter's role in simultaneous talk in interpreted interaction. Multilingua 12(4): 341–363.

Ruben RJ, Schwartz R (1999) Necessity versus sufficiency: the role of input in language acquisition. International Journal of Pediatric Otorhinolaryngology 15–47(2):137–140.

Rudduck J, Hopkins D (eds) (1985) Research as a Basis for Teaching. London: Heinemann.

Sacks H (1995 [1968]) Second stories; ' Mm hm'; Story prefaces; 'Local news'; Tellability. In Jefferson G (ed) Harvey Sacks. Lectures on Conversation, Vol. II, Part I, Lecture 1. Oxford: Basil Blackwell.

Sacks H, Schegloff EA, Jefferson G (1974) A simplest systematics for the organisation of turn-taking in conversation. Language 50(4): 696–735.

Sanderson G (1997) Developing your own IEP. Paper given at the National Educational Interpreters Conference, Long Beach, CA, 3 August 1997.

Saur R, Popp-Stone MJ, Hurley-Lawrence E (1987) The classroom participation of mainstreamed hearing impaired college students. Volta Review 89 (6) 277–286.

Saxton M, Gallaway C (1998). Acquiring the grammatical system: how do children recover from their errors. Deafness and Education (Journal of the British Association of Teachers of the Deaf) 22(2): 16–23.

Schaffer HR, Liddell C (1984) Adult–child interaction under dyadic and polyadic conditions. British Journal of Developmental Psychology 2: 33–42.

Schegloff EA (1982) Discourse as interactional achievement: some uses of 'uh huh' and other things that come between sentences. In: Tannen D (ed) Analysing Discourse: text and talk. Georgetown University Round Table on Languages and Linguistics. Washington, DC: Georgetown University Press.

Schegloff EA (1984) On some questions and ambiguities in conversation. In Atkinson JM, Heritage J (eds) Structures of Social Action. Studies in Conversation Analysis. Cambridge: Cambridge University Press.

Schegloff EA (1992) Repair after next turn: the last structurally provided defence of intersubjectivity in conversation. American Journal of Sociology 97:1295–1345.

Seedhouse P (1996). Classroom interaction: possibilities and impossibilities. English Language Teaching Journal 50(1):16–25.

Seewald RC (1992) The desired sensation level method for fitting children: version 3.0. Hearing Journal 45:36–41.

Shah R (1995) The Silent Minority. London: National Children's Bureau.

Sharma A, Love D (1991) A Change in Approach. A report on the experience of Deaf People from Black and Ethnic Minority Communities. London: Royal Association in Aid of Deaf People.

Silvera M, Kapasi R (2000) Health Advocacy for Minority Ethnic Londoners: putting services on the map. London: King's Fund Publishing.

Sinclair JM, Coulthard RM (1975). Towards an Analysis of Discourse: the English used by teachers and pupils. Oxford: Oxford University Press.

Singleton JL, Supalla S, Litchfield S, Schley S (1998) From sign to word: Considering modality constraints in ASL/English bilingual education. Topics in Language Disorders 18(4): 16–29.

Siraj-Blatchford I, Clarke P (2000) Supporting Identity, Diversity and Language in the Early Years. Milton Keynes: Open University.

Snow CE (1989) Understanding social interaction and language acquisition: sentences are not enough. In: Bornstein MH, Bruner JS (eds) Interaction in Human Development. Mahwah, NJ: Lawrence Erlbaum Associates.

Snow CE (1995) Issues in the study of input: finetuning, universality, individual and developmental differences and necessary causes. In: Fletcher P, MacWhinney B (eds) The Handbook of Child Language. Oxford: Blackwell.

Spencer PE (1993) Communication behaviours of infants with hearing loss and their hearing mothers Journal of Speech and Hearing Research 36: 311–321.

Spencer PE, Meadow-Orlans KP (1996) Play, language, and maternal responsiveness: a longitudinal study of deaf and hearing infants. Child Development 67: 3176–3191.

STAR (2001) http://www.sylheti.org.uk/.

Stenhouse L (1985) Action research and the teacher's responsibility for the educational process. In: Rudduck J, Hopkins D (eds) Research as a Basis for Teaching. London: Heinemann.

Stinson M, Lang H (1994) The potential impact on deaf students of the full inclusion movement. In: Johnson R, Cohen O (eds) Implications and Complications for Deaf Students of the Full Inclusion Movement. Washington, DC: Gallaudet Research Institute.

Stinson M, Liu Y, Saur R, Long G (1996) Deaf college students' perceptions of communication in mainstream classes. Journal of Deaf Studies and Deaf Education 1(1): 40–51.

Stinson M, Stuckless ER, Henderson JB, Miller L (1988) Perceptions of hearing-impaired college students towards real-time speech-to-print. Volta Review 90: 336–348.

Storkey M (1994) London's Ethnic Minorities. One city, many communities. An analysis of the 1991 Census results. London: London Research Centre.

Strapp CM (1999) Mothers', fathers', and siblings' responses to children's language errors: comparing sources of negative evidence. Journal of Child Language 26: 373–391.

Stubbs M (1990) Language, Schools and Classrooms, 2nd edn. London: Routledge.

Stuckless ER (1983) Real-time transliteration of speech into print for hearing-impaired students in regular classes. American Annals of the Deaf 16: 619–624.

Supalla SJ (1990–1991) Manually coded English: the modality question in signed language development. In: Siple P, Fischer SD (eds) Theoretical Issues in Sign Language Research. Chicago, IL: University of Chicago Press.

Sutherland H (1994) Bilingual initiatives for sign at home and school. In Kyle JG (ed) Growing Up In Sign and Word. University of Bristol: Centre for Deaf Studies.

Sutherland H, Kyle J (1993) Deaf Children at Home, Final Report. University of Bristol: Centre for Deaf Studies.

Sutton GJ, Rowe SJ (1997) Risk factors for childhood sensori-neural hearing loss in the Oxford Region. British Journal of Audiology 31:39–54.

Svartholm K (1993) Bilingual education for the deaf in Sweden. Sign Language Studies 81: 291–332.

Svirsky MA, Robbins AM, Kirk KI, Pisoni DB, Miyamoto RT (2000) Language development in profoundly deaf children with cochlear implants. Psychological Science 11(2): 153–158.

Swain M (2000) The output hypothesis and beyond: mediating acquisition through collaborative dialogue. In: Lantolf JP (ed) Socio-cultural Theory and Second Language Learning. Oxford: Oxford University Press.

Swanwick R (2001) The demands of a sign context for bilingual teachers and learners: an observation of language use and learning experiences. Deafness and Education International 3(2): 62–79.

Tait M, Lutman ME, Nikolopoulos TP (2001) Communication development in young deaf children: review of the video analysis method. International Journal of Pediatric Otorhinolaryngology 61: 105–112.

Tait M, Lutman ME, Robinson K (2000) Preimplant measures of preverbal communicative behavior as predictors of cochlear implant outcomes in children. Ear and Hearing 21(1): 18–24.

Tait M, Nikolopoulos TP, Lutman ME, Wilson D, Wells P (2001) Video analysis of preverbal communication behaviours: use and reliability. Deafness and Education International 3(1): 38–43.

Takala M, Kuusela J, Takala E (2000) A good future for deaf children: a five-year sign language intervention project. American Annals of the Deaf 145(4): 366–374.

Tarplee C (1996) Working on young children's utterances: prosodic aspects of repetition during picture labelling. In: Couper-Kuhlen E, Selting M (eds) Prosody in Conversation Interactional Studies. Cambridge: Cambridge University Press.

Tate G, Collins J, Tymms P (2001) Assessments using BSL: Issues of translation for performance indicators in primary schools. Unpublished paper CEM Centre, University of Durham. Presented at BERA conference, Leeds, 2001.

Tharp R, Gallimore R (1991) A theory of teaching as assisted performance. In: Light P, Sheldon S, Woodhead M (eds) (1991) Learning to Think. London: Routledge.

Thornbury S (1996) Teachers research teacher talk. English Language Teaching Journal 50(4): 279–289.

Tomasello M, Conti-Ramsden G, Ewert B (1990) Young children's conversations with their mothers and fathers: differences in breakdown and repair. Journal of Child Language 17: 115–130.

Tomasello M, Mannle S (1985) Pragmatics of sibling speech to 1-year-olds. Child Development 56: 911–917.

Tomblin JB, Spencer L, Flock S, Tyler R, Gantz B (1999) A comparison of language achievement in children with cochlear implants and children using hearing aids. Journal of Speech, Language and Hearing Research 42: 497–511.

Tremblay-Leveau H, Leclerc S, Nadel J (1999) Linguistic skills of 16- and 23-month-old twins and singletons in a triadic context. First Language 19: 233–254.

Tucker I, Powell C (1991) The Hearing Impaired Child and School. London: Souvenir Press.

Turner S (1996) Meeting the needs of children under five with sensori-neural hearing loss from ethnic minority families. Journal of the British Association of Teachers of the Deaf 20(4): 91–100.

Tymms P (1999) Baseline Assessment and Monitoring in Primary Schools: Achievements, Attitudes and Value-added Indicators. London: David Fulton Publishers.

Tymms P, Albone S (2002) Performance indicators in primary schools. In: Visscher A, Coe R (eds) School Improvement Through Performance Feedback. Lisse: Swets and Zeitlinger.

Tymms P, Brien D, Merrell C, Collins J, Jones P (2000) Young Deaf Children and the Prediction of reading and maths. Unpublished paper, CEM Centre, University of Durham. Presented at BERA conference, Cardiff, 2000.

Uzawa K (1996) Second language learner's processes of L1 writing, L2 writing and translation from L1 into L2. Journal of Second Language Writing 5(3): 271–294.

Vaccari C, Marschark M (1997) Communication between parents and deaf children: implications for social-emotional development. Journal of Child Psychology and Psychiatry 38(7): 793–801.

Valero Garcia J (1999) Teaching Conversational Control to Deaf Students. Mimeographed Paper. Faculty of Psychology, Universitat Autonoma de Barcelona, Barcelona, Spain.

Van der Lem T (1987) An early intervention programme. In: Kyle J (ed.) Sign and School. Clevedon: Multilingual Matters.

Vandell DL, Wilson KS (1987) Infants' interactions with mother, sibling and peer: contrasts and relations between interaction systems. Child Development 58: 176–186.

Vanniasegaram I, Tungland OP, Bellman S (1993) A five-year review of children with deafness in a multiethnic community. Journal of Audiological Medicine 2: 9–19.

Vidas S, Hassan R, Parnes LS (1992) Real-life performance considerations of four paediatric multichannel cochlear implant recipients. Journal of Otolaryngology 21: 387–393.

Vygotsky LS (1978) Mind in Society: The Development of Higher Psychological Processes. Cambridge, MA: Harvard University Press.

Walker LM (1993) Academic learning in an integrated setting for hearing impaired students: A description of an Australian unit's efforts to meet the challenge. Volta Review 95(3): 295–304.

Waltzman SB, Cohen NL (1998) Cochlear implantation in children younger than 2 years old. American Journal of Otology 19: 158–162.

Waltzman SB, Cohen NL, Gomolin RH, Green JE, Shapiro WH, Hoffman RA, Roland JT (1997) Open-set speech perception in congenitally deaf children using cochlear implants. American Journal of Otology 18: 342–349.

Watkins S, Pitman P, Walden B (1998) The deaf mentor experimental project for young children who are deaf and their families. American Annals of the Deaf 143: 29–34.

Watson L (1998) Oralism – current policy and practice. In: Gregory S, Knight P, McCracken W, Powers S, Watson L (eds) Issues in Deaf Education. London: David Fulton.

Watson L, Parsons J (1998) Supporting deaf pupils in mainstream settings. In: Gregory S, Knight P, McCracken W, Powers S, Watson L (eds) Issues in Deaf Education. London: David Fulton.

Webster A, Heineman-Gosschalk R (2000) Deaf children's encounters with written texts: contrasts between hearing teachers and deaf adults in supporting reading. Deafness and Education International 2(2): 26–44.

Webster A (1986) Deafness, Development and Literacy. London: Methuen.

Wells G (1993) Re-evaluating the IRF sequence: A proposal for the articulation of theories of activity and discourse for the analysis of teaching and learning in the classroom. Linguistics and Education 5: 1–37.

Wilbur R (2000) The use of ASL to support the development of English and literacy. Journal of Deaf Studies and Deaf Education 5(1): 81–104.

Willes M (1981). Learning to take part in classroom interaction. In: French P, MacLure M (eds) Adult-Child Conversation. London: Croom Helm.

Williams CN (1994) A 'real life' clinical trial approach opens new avenues of hearing care. Hearing Instruments 45: 13–15.

Winston E (1989) Transliteration, what's the message? In: Lucas C (ed) The Sociolinguistics of the Deaf Community. Washington, DC: Gallaudet University, pp. 147–164.

Winston E (1994) An interpreted education: inclusion or exclusion? In: Johnson RC, Cohen OP (eds) Implications and Complications for Deaf Students of the Full Inclusion Movement. Gallaudet Research Institute Occasional Paper 94-2. Washington, DC: Gallaudet University.

Winston E (1997) Interpreting in the classroom: providing accessibility or creating new barriers. Notes from a lecture given at the National Educational Interpreters Conference, Long Beach, California, 3 August 1997.

Winter K (1998) Speech and language provision for bilingual children: aspects of current service. International Journal of Language and Communication Disorders 34(1): 85–98.

Woll B (1998) Development of signed and spoken languages. In: Gregory S, Knight P, McCracken W, Powers S, Watson L (eds) Issues in Deaf Education. London: David Fulton Publishers.

Wood DJ (1988) How Children Think and Learn: the social contexts of cognitive development. Oxford: Blackwell.

Wood DJ (1991) Aspects of teaching and learning. In: Light P, Sheldon S, Woodhead M (eds) Learning to Think. London: Routledge.

Wood DJ (1992) Teaching talk. In: Norman, K (ed.) Thinking Voices: the work of the National Oracy Project. London: Hodder and Stoughton.

Wood DJ (1998) How Children Think and Learn: the social contexts of cognitive development, 2nd edn. Oxford: Blackwell.

Wood DJ, O'Malley C (1996) Collaborative learning between peers: an overview. Educational Psychology in Practice 11: 4–9.

Wood DJ, Bruner JS, Ross G (1976) The role of tutoring in problem solving. Journal of Child Psychology and Psychiatry and Allied Disciplines 17: 89–100.

Wood DJ, Wood HA, Middleton D (1978) An experimental evaluation of four face-to-face teaching strategies. International Journal of Behavioral Development 1: 131–147.

Wood DJ, Wood HA, Ainsworth S, O'Malley C (1995) On becoming a tutor: Toward an ontogenetic model. Cognition and Instruction 13: 565–581.

Wood DJ, Wood HA, Griffiths AJ, Howarth CI (1986) Teaching and Talking with Deaf Children. Chichester: Wiley.

Wood HA, Wood DJ (1984). An experimental evaluation of the effects of five styles of communication on the language of hearing impaired children. Journal of Child Psychology and Psychiatry 21(1): 45–62.

Wood PL, Kyle JG (1989) Hi Linc: computer note-taking and transcription for deaf people. Leverhulme Trust report, unpublished paper, Centre for Deaf Studies, Bristol.

Woodward JC (1972) Implications for sociolinguistic research amongst the deaf. Sign Language Studies 1:1–7.

Woolfe T, Want SC, Siegal M (2002) Signposts to development: theory of mind in deaf children. Child Development 73 (3): 768–778.

Woollett A (1986) The influence of older siblings on the language environment of young children. British Journal of Developmental Psychology 4:235–245.

Yin RK (1989) Case Study Research: Design and Methods, 2nd edn. London: Sage.

Yoshinaga-Itano C, Snyder L (1985) Form and meaning in the written language of hearing-impaired children. Volta Review 87: 75–90.

Youdelman K, Messerly C (1996) Computer-assisted note-taking for mainstreamed hearing-impaired students. Volta Review 98(4): 191–199.

Young AM (1997) Conceptualising parents' sign language use in bilingual early intervention. Journal of Deaf Studies and Deaf Education 2(4): 264–276.

Young AM (2001) The implementation of universal neonatal hearing screening (UNHS): lessons from developments in the USA, Chapter 7 (available on: *http://www.deafnessatbirth.org.uk*).

Young AM, Andrews E (2001) Parents' experiences of universal neonatal hearing screening: a Critical review of the literature and its implications for the implementation of new UNHS programs. Journal of Deaf Studies and Deaf Education 6(3) 149–160.

Young AM, Ackerman J, Kyle J (1998) Looking On: deaf people and the organisation of services. Bristol: The Policy Press.

Young AM, Clibben J, Sutherland H (forthcoming) Family intervention services employing D/deaf adults – a systematic review of the literature.

Young AM, Griggs M., Sutherland H (2000) Deaf Child and Family Intervention Services Using Deaf Adult Role Models: a national survey of development, practice and progress. London: Royal National Institute for Deaf People.

Young AM, Huntington A (2002) Working with Deaf Babies from Birth to Two in Light of the Children Act 1989 (available on: *http://www.deafnessatbirth.org.uk*).

Young AM, Sutherland H, Griggs M (1999) The Language Link Project – An Evaluation. London: Royal National Institute for Deaf People.

Zimmerman-Phillips S, Osberger MJ, Robbins AM (1997) Infant–Toddler Meaningful Auditory Integration Scale (IT-MAIS). Synlar: Advanced Bionic Corporation.

Useful websites

C-Print in Further Education
http://www.rit.edu/~easi/itd/itdv01n2/cuddihy.html

Current developments in Automatic Speech Recognition and deaf education   *http://netac.rit.edu/publication/asr.html*

Deafness @ birth to 2   *http://www.deafnessatbirth.org.uk*

DfEE. Ethnic Minority Achievement and Traveller Children Achievement Grant   *http://www.dfee.gov.uk/ethnic/guide.htm*

DfEE. National Literacy Strategy
http://vtc.ngfl.gov.uk/literacy/nls/eal.html

Direct Learning   *http://www.directlearn.co.uk/deafres.htm*

The Incredible Years   *http://www.incredibleyears.com*

National Association for Language Development in the Curriculum (NALDIC)   *http://www.naldic.org.uk/*

National Deaf Children's Society (NDCS)   *http://www.ndcs.org.uk*

Newborn Hearing Screening Programme   *http://www.unhs.org.uk*

Office of National Statistics
http://www.statistics.gov.uk/statbase/xsdataset.asp

Performance Indicators in Primary Schools (PIPS)
http://www.cem.dur.ac.uk/pips

Qualifications and Curriculum Authority. Key Skills
http://www.qca.org.uk/nq/ks/com_app_it2.asp

Qualifications and Curriculum Authority. Special arrangements for the
tests   *http://www.qca.org.uk/ca/tests/ara/ks2_special.asp*

Royal National Institute for Deaf People (RNID)
http://www.rnid.org.uk

STAR   *http://www.sylheti.org.uk/*

Author index

Subject index